Mattering

Mattering

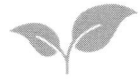

*The Secret to Building a Life of
Deep Connection and Purpose*

Jennifer Breheny Wallace

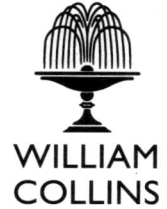

**WILLIAM
COLLINS**

William Collins
An imprint of HarperCollins*Publishers*
1 London Bridge Street
London SE1 9GF

WilliamCollinsBooks.com

HarperCollins*Publishers*
Macken House, 39/40 Mayor Street Upper
Dublin 1, D01 C9W8, Ireland

First published in Great Britain in 2026 by William Collins

First published in the United States by Portfolio / Penguin, an imprint of Penguin
Random House LLC in 2026

1

A catalogue record for this book is available from the British Library

ISBN 978-0-00-871882-4 (hardback)
ISBN 978-0-00-871883-1 (trade paperback)

Grateful acknowledgement is made for permission to reprint an excerpt
from *Wild Hope* by Donna Ashworth, first published by Black & White
Publishing London, an imprint of Bonnier Books UK Limited.

Book design by Alissa Rose Theodor

Printed and bound in the UK using 100% Renewable
Electricity at CPI Group (UK) Ltd

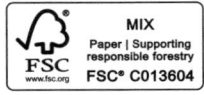

To my husband, Peter, our family, and friends—
my truest teachers of mattering

I don't want to end up simply having visited this world.

—Mary Oliver, "When Death Comes"

Contents

Introduction   The Mattering Core   1

1   Connect to Your Impact   15

2   The Good Kind of Weight   35

3   Mattering Too Much   59

4   Everyone Needs (to Be) a Cornerman   91

5   Tuning In   121

6   When the Rug Gets Pulled:
        Coping with Life's Transitions   145

7   How We Spend Our Days: Mattering at Work   173

8   Be an Architect: Mattering Spaces   203

Epilogue   The Power of "We Matter"   227

Acknowledgments   233
Appendix: Mattering Assessment   237
Notes   241
Index   259

Author's Note

Due to the sensitive nature of these conversations, some names and identifying details have been changed. In those cases, I included only a first name. Everyone identified with a full name chose to be named.

Mattering

The Mattering Core

I t began with a clementine.

As I arrived at the Harlem train station one early fall morning, the space was already buzzing with activity. Commuters rushed past each other, train brakes screeched on the tracks, and the air smelled of a mix of freshly brewed coffee and diesel fumes from the old trains running up above. Tucked away in the corner of the station was a brightly lit bodega.

Though small, the space felt abundant: The neatly organized shelves brimmed with snacks, bottled water lined the refrigerator, and colorful fruit spilled from decorative wicker baskets. A man with gray hair called to me from behind the counter. "Ah, welcome," he said. "It's wonderful to see you." He spoke with the warmth of someone greeting a regular, though I wasn't. As I browsed, I overheard his conversation with another customer, someone who clearly *was* a regular, about the clementines he had picked up at the market that morning. "I remembered how much you liked them last time," the shopkeeper said. "When I saw them,

I knew I had to bring them in again for you." The customer thanked him for always being so kind and thoughtful.

Those clementines had caught my eye, too, their bright skins a welcome contrast to the station's muted gray. But what stayed with me as I took the train out of town was the care in the exchange, the way the shopkeeper's thoughtfulness did more than offer fruit. It was a sign that someone had paid attention and remembered, proof of connection in a world that often feels indifferent. A small gesture that said: *You matter.*

Later that day, as I boarded the train back to New York, the car was crowded with commuters settling into their seats. I pulled out the last of the clementines from the bodega and began peeling one as juice squirted everywhere. Suddenly, a young man in his early twenties stormed into the car. His eyes darted around, and his chest heaved with visible anger. He shouted, startling everyone. From what I could gather, he'd had words with someone on the platform. The other person was gone, but his anger remained.

As he yelled, the other passengers averted their gazes and lowered into their seats, maybe out of fear of what might happen, but also maybe because his desperation was too much to witness. Quickly and calmly, a conductor approached the man. He didn't issue threats, bark orders, or try to overpower him. Instead, he spoke softly, asking if everything was okay or if he needed anything. Then he pointed out an open chair and gently asked the man for his ticket. Despite being considerably shorter, the conductor had a grounding effect on the man. The interaction was masterful to witness. What could have escalated into something more dangerous had been resolved through respect and compassion.

Once the train car was calm, I stared out the window, thinking about what I had just seen. It struck me how the young man, so consumed by rage, softened at the conductor's words. The conductor could have thrown him off the train for being disruptive, but that's not what happened. Instead, the conductor engaged with him as a person worthy of dignity.

At the time, I was deep into researching *Never Enough*, my book about how our culture of achievement is driving a mental health crisis among adolescents. One idea kept surfacing: mattering—the feeling that we are valued and needed by others. Again and again, I found that the kids who were thriving shared one thing in common: that they felt they mattered for who they were deep at their core. Mattering acted as a kind of protective shield that buffered against anxiety and depression. But what I saw on that train clarified something else. Mattering isn't just for young people. It's for everyone, everywhere. While I understood the concept intellectually, that moment on the train made it visceral. Adults crave the same recognition, the same sense of being seen and valued. I felt it in the bodega owner's warmth. I heard it in the conductor's voice, how he looked past the young man's rage and spoke to the person beneath it.

Slowly, it became clear to me. The man on the train wasn't just lashing out. He was reaching out. In his own confused, chaotic way, he was begging the world to answer our most fundamental human questions: *Do you see me? Do you hear me? Do I matter?*

The conductor answered him with compassion and care.

Our universal need to matter

Since that day, I've been on a journey—part pilgrimage, part investigation—to uncover what makes us feel like we matter and what makes that feeling vanish, even in lives that look full from the outside. Psychologists, sociologists, and philosophers vary in their definitions of mattering, but at its core, mattering is the feeling that we are valued and have value to add to the world.

> **Feeling Valued + Adding Value = Mattering**

Mattering is the assurance that our presence and actions are significant to others. It's the pull you feel toward someone who genuinely appreciates you and your input, or the warm feeling you get when you see that your efforts have made a difference. It's knowing others rely on you in big and small ways. It is the meaningful way we fit into each other's lives and the wider world, like essential pieces of a puzzle.

On the surface, mattering may seem simple. But dig a little deeper, and it speaks to the most profound complexities of the human experience. Mattering is the story we tell ourselves about our place in the world, as in, Do people value and appreciate me—or do I go unnoticed? Do I truly belong, or am I moving through the world alone? Does my life make a difference to others, or would it not matter if I weren't here?

It was legendary sociologist Morris Rosenberg who first introduced the idea of mattering in the 1980s. Since then, the concept has slowly evolved, spanning new disciplines. In recent years, the idea has gained fresh traction among researchers and practitioners alike. As rates of anxiety, burnout, and disconnection have surged, scholars in fields as varied as neuroscience, workplace culture, education, and public health are turning to mattering to better understand what people need to thrive. It is emerging as one of the most essential, yet overlooked, pillars of well-being.

Mattering is what psychologists call a "meta-need" or "umbrella term" because part of its power lies in how it encompasses familiar concepts—feelings of connection, belonging, and purpose—under a single, intuitive concept. In fact, what makes it particularly powerful is that it transcends these individual concepts. For example, mattering goes deeper than belonging: You can belong to a group, such as a workplace, a classroom, or a family, but not feel like you matter to the group. Similarly, mattering goes deeper than purpose: You can have a sense of meaning in your work, community, or relationships, but mattering means you also know your actions and efforts make a positive impact on those around you.

Mattering is so deeply ingrained in us that after basic survival needs like food and shelter are met, it is the need to matter that drives human behavior. We long to feel valued by our family, friends, and community and to add value in return, to make a positive impact and contribute meaningfully to the lives of others. That motivation is part of our evolutionary inheritance. For our earliest ancestors, being valued by the group meant support and protection from danger. To be ignored or cast out was a threat to survival itself. That primal fear and longing are still wired in us today.

We may not have always used the word "mattering," but the need is as old as humanity itself. Psychologists, philosophers, and spiritual leaders across time have been trying to name this need, trying to understand what it means to truly belong and make a difference. We find it in the writings of Aristotle, who wrote that *eudaimonia*, the flourishing life, was achievable through developing and exercising virtues such as generosity and friendship within a community. It is at the heart of our most familiar psychological theories, such as Alfred Adler's assertion that contributing meaningfully to others is foundational for well-being.

It appears in the teachings of religion. For example, in Judaism and Christianity, the idea that each individual is "made in the image of God" (*imago Dei*) underscores intrinsic worth. Islam similarly teaches that each person is endowed with dignity (*karama*) by their Creator. Hinduism speaks of the divine spark (*atman*) within every being, while Buddhism's emphasis on interconnectedness suggests that each life inherently affects the whole. Across traditions, the message is clear that every person matters.

Rituals designed to make individuals feel valued, from coming-of-age ceremonies to retirement celebrations, are woven into daily life. These "mattering practices" offer a sense of belonging and purpose and remind participants that their existence holds meaning. The universal need to matter connects us all whether we are young or old, rich or poor, introverts or extroverts, caregivers or leaders. It transcends identity, profession, background, and belief, reminding us that for all our differences, we are united by the same need to feel valued, to be needed, and to know that our presence leaves a mark on the world.

When I first heard about the concept of mattering while researching my first book, *Never Enough*, I immediately felt a transcendent understanding of the concept. It was like someone turned on a light and gave a name to something I'd been circling for years without quite landing on—one of those rare moments when a single word unlocks a whole universe of meaning. The concept felt both startlingly new and instantly familiar.

"Mattering," I thought, "is what life is all about."

The longer I sat with the concept, the more its power revealed itself. *Mattering* gives language to those unmistakably good moments, like when someone remembers your name, when your child repeats something you once taught them, or when a friend's face lights up simply because you walked into the room. Just as striking, it also names what feels so painfully absent in our world today. Could a lack of mattering be at the root of some of our most personal struggles—feeling burned out or invisible at work, unheard in our relationships, or irrelevant in our communities?

The modern mattering crisis

In the six years I spent researching mattering, I've asked hundreds of people around the world this question: *Do you feel like you matter?* Across industries and ideologies, across age, class, and geography, too often the answer was "no" or "not anymore." One parent described feeling invisible because her needs came after everyone else's. A doctor told me how powerless she felt when insurance companies dismissed her years of training and denied her patients the care she knew they needed. An executive, nearing retirement, worried about becoming irrelevant once he stopped working. A college student told me she only felt like she mattered when her grades were high and her weight was low. A mother of three grown children, once the center of their world, told me she no longer felt she had a place in it. An elderly man said the hardest part of aging was that no one relied on him anymore.

Each conversation left me with more urgent questions. They also made me think about my own life and the people in it in a new way. Soon, my children will be grown and flown. How will I protect my mattering during that seismic shift? How will I support theirs? Friends confided that they were feeling unappreciated at work. Others who had stepped away from careers to raise their kids were wrestling with a loss of identity and purpose. Everywhere I looked, people were grappling with this erosion of mattering, whether it was not feeling valued or no longer feeling like they had a chance to add meaningful value in this world. Even headlines started to read differently to me: "Men Are in a Loneliness Epidemic," "Why So Many Employees Are 'Quiet Quitting,'" and "The Caregiver Crisis."

> **Mattering is double-edged—powerful when we feel it and destructive when we don't.**

The deep sense of crisis we are feeling globally, marked by rising rates of depression, loneliness, and burnout, has been blamed on many factors, such as polarized politics, rapid technological advances, social media, and culture wars. Caregivers are overwhelmed by the mental and emotional labor of holding their families together, often while working full-time. Men are no longer sure where or how they fit into society. Workplaces are more demanding than ever and less fulfilling, and on top of that, AI is now coming for our jobs. Our faith in government institutions has eroded, so we don't believe that any relief or remedy is on the way. Many people have turned away from religion and the community it offers. Technology has eliminated in-person interaction, third spaces have disappeared, and trust in our neighbors has crumbled.

These widespread struggles, and the effects they've had on all of us, from isolation to exhaustion to a persistent sense of instability, can also be understood as symptoms of not feeling seen, not feeling valued, and not feeling essential. We're uncertain whether what we do makes any real difference. We don't feel needed, at least not in the ways that sustain us. The inequality we see, the grind we can't escape, and the disconnection from institutions and each other all chip away at our belief that we are valuable. That we *add* value. That our presence matters.

Mental health struggles often correlate with feeling invisible or unimportant, serving as stark indicators that mattering is missing. This absence is at the heart of a troubling shift. Since 2014, US life expectancy has been declining, reversing decades of progress. A major driver of this trend is what sociologists call "deaths of despair"—suicides, overdoses, and alcohol-related deaths—fueled by rising loneliness, disconnection, and job loss. Globally, nearly one in four people, over a billion, report feeling very or fairly lonely, according to a 2023 survey across 140 countries.

Mattering is like gravity: unseen but essential. It holds us in place. It steadies us. When we feel that we matter, we feel anchored. When it's missing, we begin to drift. We lose our footing and our sense of where we fit. The world feels colder, unwelcoming. The human brain wasn't built for this kind of world. We often describe what's happening around us as a mental health crisis, but this language only provides a partial picture. In truth, we are living through a *social* health crisis, a profound breakdown of the relationships that once protected us. We've lost track of our most basic human needs for connection and contribution. Now we often feel tempted to fill that void with counterfeit forms of mattering—chasing attention over connection, prestige over purpose, and money over meaning. The rise in loneliness, burnout, and anxiety is the predictable consequence of a society that has forgotten how to make people feel valued.

At its most extreme, the belief that we fundamentally do not matter is what psychologist Gordon Flett has termed "anti-mattering." If mattering is what makes life feel significant, then anti-mattering is its converse, the profoundly painful feeling that we are invisible, inconsequential. Anti-mattering is distinct from the passing moments when we question our worth, like feeling overlooked in a team meeting or realizing a friend didn't invite us to a group dinner. These are everyday human experiences, and though they may sting, they tend to fade with time or reassurance. Anti-mattering, by contrast, is more enduring and more corrosive. It's the gnawing belief that we don't matter to anyone. If allowed to fester, anti-mattering exacts a profound toll.

> *The worst sin towards our fellow creatures is not to hate them, but to be indifferent to them: that's the essence of inhumanity.*
>
> —George Bernard Shaw

When we fail to meet this need, when we allow people to move through the world feeling unseen, unwanted, and unneeded, we court dangerous consequences. Individuals who go on to commit heinous acts are not necessarily born that way. Often, they are profoundly isolated and feel invisible, with no one depending on them, noticing their presence or absence, or thinking much about them. In such a void, some people will lash out, seeking negative attention to prove that they can make an impact, as in "I'll show you I matter." Others may turn against themselves, reach for substances, or self-harm to try to escape the psychic pain. The more I learned about mattering, the more convinced I became that it's more than a feel-good concept or abstract academic theory—it is a societal imperative.

The mattering core

In a world that can leave us feeling invisible, disconnected, and purposeless, I kept wondering: *Who's thriving? What do they have that others don't?* What I found is that the people who are doing well have built what I call a "mattering core": a sturdy, internal sense of feeling valued by family, friends, colleagues, and their community, and knowing how they add value back. Think of the mattering core as a kind of internal infrastructure. When life gets hard and we feel lost, invisible, or worn down, we can return to this core to steady us. It reminds us who we are and why we are valued. And here's the best part: This core isn't fixed. We can strengthen it in ourselves and the people we care about in our homes, communities, and workplaces. Mattering is a practice, a foundation, a way forward.

When we have a strong mattering core, we feel more grounded and resilient. It connects us to the best in ourselves and others, and it invites us to know one another more deeply. In our relationships, mattering gives us the words to express how much we value one another and the practices to sustain those bonds. At work, we're less likely to burn out because we know that what we do makes a difference. At a societal level, mattering offers a shared framework for understanding the roots of disconnection and suffering as well as the conditions that allow people to thrive. Reclaiming and rebuilding mattering is both a personal goal and a collective call to action for creating the kind of world we so desperately need. We need a new architecture for how we live and work and love—a social intervention—and that's precisely what the framework of mattering offers us.

As I stepped off the train and made my way home, I couldn't stop thinking about the conductor and the young man and the shopkeeper at the bodega. I was struck by how the smallest moments could say, *I see you. You matter*—and how starved so many of us are to feel that way. This crisis of mattering began to feel to me like an emergency. That night, I made a promise to follow this thread of mattering wherever it took me.

This book is the result of everything I've learned.

If you feel invisible or burned out at work, this book is for you. If your children are grown and you're left wondering where you now fit in their world, or if you're deep in the chaos of parenthood, so overextended that your own needs barely register—this is for you, too. If you've just relocated and your social network has vanished; if you're living with chronic illness and feel like the world has moved on without you; if you're watching someone you love drift—an adult child, a partner, a friend, an aging parent—or if everything looks fine on the outside but inside you feel aimless and disconnected, this book is for you. Whatever your story, the ache is the same: *Do I matter? Will I ever feel that I matter again?*

Together, we'll explore how to foster mattering in ourselves and those we care about at home, at work, and in our wider world—and how to cope when we feel like we don't. To start, we'll unpack the essential elements of what I call the mattering core: how to recognize your impact, why it's vital to feel relied upon (but not too much), and what happens when others attune to your inner world and invest in you. These core elements help fortify our everyday lives and build stronger relationships. Next, we'll look at how life's transitions can shake our sense of mattering and how we can rebuild it in new ways. Finally, we'll turn outward to the larger world, examining how mattering can be cultivated in our workplaces and communities. In each chapter, you'll meet people whose stories of mattering lost and regained moved me so deeply that I had to share them with you, alongside simple, actionable practices to help you build a life that feels more connected, more purposeful, and more deeply lived.

So come with me. Let's begin.

The Mattering Core

Recognition: You and your actions are valued, and your absence would be felt.

Reliance: You feel needed because others depend on you.

Importance: You feel significant because you're prioritized.

Ego Extension: You feel cared for because others are invested in your well-being.

Attunement: You feel deeply understood and meaningfully responded to.

In the appendix, you'll find a series of statements to reflect on. You might consider visiting that reflection exercise now, and then again after you read the book, to see how your sense of mattering evolves as you learn more about the concept.

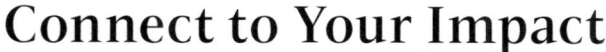

CHAPTER 1

Connect to Your Impact

The Mattering Core

Recognition: You and your actions are valued, and your absence would be felt.

Reliance: You feel needed because others depend on you.

Importance: You feel significant because you're prioritized.

Ego Extension: You feel cared for because others are invested in your well-being.

Attunement: You feel deeply understood and meaningfully responded to.

Greg Bulanow felt glass crunch beneath his boots as he rushed toward the wreck. It was one of his first calls as a rookie firefighter, and he knew every minute counted. The driver was alive but trapped under the twisted steel. Greg's training took over. He squeezed through a jagged opening to reach the woman, who was crying out in pain. Her breathing was quick and panicked. Greg spoke to her gently. "We're going to get you out of here," he promised as he draped his heavy bunker coat around the woman to shield her from the flying shards of metal and glass as they worked to free her. Greg stayed by her side, steadying her through every jolt. When the last barrier gave way and she was lifted to safety, Greg felt both drained and deeply grateful. He had helped someone through one of the worst moments of their life.

Greg never planned to become a firefighter. After earning an English degree from a small liberal arts college in Ohio, he moved to Charleston, South Carolina, with his new wife, Jacqueline, envisioning a life of cobblestone streets and a future in writing. He'd work for a year or two, then pursue an MFA in creative writing. When he saw a fire department job listing in the newspaper, he applied, thinking it would be a way to save money, have an adventure, and collect good stories for graduate school.

But around the time Greg helped extract the woman from the wreck, his view of firefighting began to change. He was thinking less about becoming a writer and more about the meaning he found in the work. When Greg and his crew arrived on the scene of a medical emergency or accident, there was a moment when everything shifted. Strangers handed over their loved ones with absolute trust, believing that Greg and his team would make things better. And Greg wanted to live up to that trust. Over the next decade, his dedication paid off. By age thirty-six, he was chief of the North Charleston Fire Department, overseeing 250 employees across eleven stations.

But once Greg stepped into his new leadership role, firefighter morale—a perennial problem—now became his responsibility. The demands of the work were relentless. These men and women responded to roughly twenty-two thousand calls a year, and the physical and emotional signs of burnout were hard to miss. Many firefighters felt upper management did not understand their day-to-day challenges. Camaraderie was fading, and their personal lives seemed to be suffering, too. Some firefighters had gone through multiple divorces, while others were turning to heavy drinking. Firefighters were leaving the department, and the constant turnover left Greg scrambling to fill station gaps. Greg attempted to rebuild morale with new trucks and top-of-the-line gear and equipment. But when he unveiled the improvements, he was met with skepticism. Someone muttered that the department was trying to buy their support. The comment stung. It also made Greg realize that the problem needed a deeper solution.

The problem of invisibility

We live in a culture that constantly tells us that the answer to discontent is to find a deep, driving purpose. Self-help books, commencement speeches, and social media posts urge us to discover our calling, align our work with our values, raise children with intention, or serve the world through volunteering. This emphasis on meaning and purpose is understandable. It's essential to our well-being. But as I researched the burnout epidemic, the advice to "do something meaningful" often fell short. Greg's firefighters were a striking example. These were people saving lives, responding to emergencies, and doing work most would call deeply meaningful. And yet, many of them were burned out or disengaged, with some even leaving the force. It didn't add up.

When I asked Greg about this paradox, his response surprised me. He explained that firefighters can sometimes struggle to see the impact of their work. My head tilted, confused. *Wait—they literally save lives—how is that even possible?* Greg then explained something I didn't know. Firefighters are often the first to arrive at a crisis, whether it's a multicar pileup on the interstate or a heart attack in the middle of the night. After firefighters pull people out of burning cars or revive someone, the paramedics or ER staff take over. The patients are whisked to the hospital, while the firefighters pack up their equipment, climb into the truck, and head back to the station. Usually, they never hear how things turn out, Greg said. They never learn, for instance, whether the woman they helped rescue from the car wreck made it to the hospital or ever walked again—if their efforts that night made any difference. This uncertainty wears on them. There's no closure, no connection to the outcome. Instead, they just write up their report and then head out to the next call. Greg told me that, over time, the lack of closure can erode morale and contribute to burnout or mental health struggles.

> *There's a common denominator in the human experience that we all share. We all want to know that what we do, what we say, and who we are matters. . . . Every argument is really about, Do you see me? Do you see me? Does what I say mean anything to you? Do I matter to you?*
>
> —Oprah Winfrey

This disconnection from our impact isn't only a problem of workplaces. So often, we move through our days unsure if what we do matters to anyone at all. Like firefighters, we often struggle not because we don't contribute, but because we rarely see the impact. We drop off soup for a sick friend but never hear whether it brought comfort. We contribute to a GoFundMe, uncertain if our donation helped. We give advice to an acquaintance preparing for a job interview and never hear how it went. Whether it's because we live in a culture that prizes self-sufficiency or simply because we are busy and distracted, too often we forget to close the loop with others. Over time, this lack of closure can lead to a growing sense of detachment in our work, homes, neighborhoods, and communities.

As a rookie firefighter, Greg felt that same sense of detachment. He and his colleagues would risk their lives to put out a house fire only to pass by the same property a week later and see it demolished by the insurance company. Firefighters had risked their lives to save that house only to see it destroyed—how could that not erode morale and breed frustration?

Whether you're working in an office, managing a household, or driving a delivery route, it's difficult to stay purposeful if it seems like what you're doing has no real impact on others. When we lack the feeling that others are aware of us and our actions, we miss the very foundation of mattering, as in "the feeling that one is the object of another person's attention or notice," according to researcher Morris Rosenberg. Even small gestures of recognition, such as when a barista remembers our regular order, a colleague stops by, or a neighbor waves hello, show us that we are seen, that we hold value. Research finds these brief encounters strengthen our sense of belonging and anchor us in our communities. Similarly, we need to know that our actions make a positive impact, like a former student returning to say he pursued an advanced degree because a teacher once believed in him. In a world where much of our effort can feel invisible, these gestures become the social proof that we do, in fact, matter.

Gradually, Greg came to understand that it was exactly this kind of invisibility that had led his firefighters to feel so burned out. After the lukewarm reception to the new equipment, Greg realized what was missing. Firefighters put themselves on the line daily without seeing the lives they changed or the gratitude that often followed. Greg was determined to close that gap.

"I'm telling"

One of the first things Greg did was to direct his medical officer, the person who trains firefighters for medical calls, to begin following up on patient outcomes when firefighters requested more information. Previously, they'd often been left wondering, *Whatever happened to that little girl we pulled from the wreck?* Or, *Did the man who collapsed during his morning run survive?* Now it was the medical officer's job to find and share any available updates. Soon firefighters started receiving meaningful feedback about how their work had helped people.

Around the same time, Greg also introduced a new fire investigator, whose job was not only to determine the cause of each fire but also to debrief the crews on the efficacy of the tactics they'd used to fight it. Historically, fire investigations were kept under wraps due to the possibility of criminal inquiries, which meant firefighters rarely received feedback on whether their strategies had been effective. Just as the medical officer's follow-up system gave firefighters a clearer view of their lifesaving efforts, the fire investigator helped firefighters see that their actions directly influenced the outcome of each fire, such as saving someone's home or containing a burning building so it didn't spread to a neighbor's house, all without revealing information that would compromise an inquiry.

Greg also decided to implement a system in which, every two weeks on payday, shift commanders were required to email him at least one thing their team members had done that deserved recognition. Even if there was nothing noteworthy, they were still required to send a "nothing to report" email. This system, Greg hoped, would ensure that good work didn't go unnoticed. At first, Greg was deluged with "nothing to report" messages. Plenty of good things were happening at the fire stations, of course—acts of teamwork, lifesaving responses—but the firefighters' actions were so ingrained in the culture that people in leadership failed to notice them. Some supervisors wondered out loud why the department was thanking employees for doing what they were paid to do. "So much of being a firefighter is about action," Greg told me. "Telling people in leadership that they need to step back and observe requires a different mentality."

Recognizing that humor is a natural part of firehouse culture, where good-natured teasing helps manage stress and build camaraderie, Greg decided to shift his approach. He encouraged his firefighters to use the phrase "I'm telling" to "tattle" on one another: "I'm telling the battalion chief the great work you're doing because you deserve to be recognized for it." Perhaps the playful framing would make reporting on good work feel less like a formal obligation and more like an opportunity to joke around. The new framing steadily took root, and Greg began receiving more reports of his firefighters' admirable actions. When he received such feedback, he made it a point to respond personally by sending handwritten thank-you cards, inviting the crew to staff meetings where they were publicly praised, or presenting them with a Chief's Coin, a special token of recognition reserved for those who go above and beyond the call of duty. Once, for instance, a unit responded to a minor accident in which a car had totaled a bicycle. The cyclist was unhurt but inconsolable because her bike was her only mode of transportation, and now she would not be able to get to work. The firefighters loaded her bike onto the truck, went back to the station, repaired it, and delivered it back to her the next morning. Greg recognized their work with a Chief's Coin. This awareness, Greg knew, was the lifeblood of their purpose.

> *The deepest principle in Human Nature is the craving to be appreciated.*
>
> —William James

Gradually, Greg began to notice a shift in the firefighters. Battalion chiefs became more mindful of recognizing the daily acts of excellence that kept their teams running smoothly. Chiefs didn't wait for formal evaluations to offer feedback. A "good job" or "thanks for handling that so well" became a regular part of their communication. The firefighters were surrounded by reminders that others were aware of their actions, that they were seen, and that they mattered. At the same time, Greg also started to see signs that the firefighters' pride in their work was returning. They began to take more ownership of their stations, such as requesting new paint to create a homier environment. Some went a step further by painting murals on the walls, while others designed and printed custom T-shirts with slogans that embodied their camaraderie and expressed a renewed sense of meaning and fulfillment.

What made "I'm telling" so effective wasn't just that it surfaced good deeds; it also spotlighted the people behind them. This idea stretches beyond firehouses. In families, classrooms, offices, and friendships, people crave being seen and recognized. Research finds that when appreciation reflects the *qualities* of the person behind an action, it hits deeper. It's the difference between saying, "Thanks for staying late," and "I always know I can count on you." The first thanks them for the deed. The other affirms the doer, and it's that affirmation that connects us to our impact. Consider the difference between "Thanks for the sweater" and "You are always such a thoughtful friend." The real impact is not about the gift. It's about the thoughtfulness of the gifter.

Researchers note we often hold back from expressing appreciation because we underestimate how much it will mean or we get stuck trying to find the perfect words. That miscalculation holds us back. But it doesn't have to stop us. We can make "I'm telling" a daily habit by building in cues throughout the day to remind us. One woman I know makes a point of sending a quick note of thanks to her husband every morning on her train to work. The commute is her cue. She just drafts a short text like, "Thank you for waking up early with the kids and being such a patient and loving dad and partner." With practice, we can learn to make appreciation a reflex by starting small with just one sentence that speaks to the person behind the action.

Notice one small thing

During my first firehouse visit in South Carolina, over mugs of tea at their long kitchen table, the firefighters spoke candidly about the physical and emotional toll of their work and about the pride they felt showing up for their community, day after day. The affection they had for one another was clear. On the refrigerator hung a photo of the firefighter of the month, which was covered with playful doodles of hearts. I pointed out that the scribbles reminded me of what a high schooler might draw on her crush's yearbook photo. "Yeah, they all have a crush on me now," the honored firefighter chuckled. When I asked why the kitchen's two refrigerators were encircled with thick chains and locks, they laughed and explained. Each shift had their own refrigerator. Although they relied on each other for matters of life and death, there was no sharing of food between shifts. "You could put a stack of money on the table, and no one would touch it," one firefighter said. "Ketchup, on the other hand . . ."

When a call came in, the atmosphere in the station quickly shifted. The alarm blared, but there was no chaos, no shouting. Each firefighter knew exactly where they needed to be and what they needed to do. Helmets were grabbed, and pants and boots were quickly pulled on. Inside the truck, they handed me a headset and told me to buckle up. While we sped through the streets, lights flashing and sirens blaring, the atmosphere in the truck was focused but energized. "Hope you didn't have too much coffee this morning," one firefighter joked, gesturing at the bumps in the road that we hit with full force.

One of the calls I joined was for an electrical fire. No one was home; neighbors had called 911. Smoke billowed from the windows of the modest ranch-style house. The aluminum siding, formerly white, was streaked with black and gray. A deflated reindeer lawn ornament lay crumpled under a bush. Christmas was only two weeks away. As we pulled to a stop, the firefighters leaped into action. I watched from a safe distance as two of them rushed inside, disappearing into the dense smoke while others sprayed arcs of water at the front of the house. After about thirty minutes, the smoke subsided. When the flames were finally extinguished, I noticed two young men—the tenants who lived in the house—standing nearby, looking shocked and helpless. A firefighter noticed this, too. He turned to them, put his hand on one of their shoulders, and murmured words of comfort.

As I watched them wrap up their final checks and load the trucks, I was struck by the routine. There was no rush to celebrate or decompress. They returned to the station to prepare dinner, then got ready to do it all over again. Watching them go through the motions, I could see how easy it would be, even in extreme circumstances, to disconnect from your impact. That's why Greg's efforts to create feedback and follow-up systems were so critical. Without these reminders, even the most dedicated team could lose sight of why they ran toward danger every day.

Reflecting on this, I found myself wondering what it would look like for all of us to intentionally connect with the impact of our work. As a writer, I often spend my days alone in a room, uncertain if my words will resonate with readers. It got me thinking. If we could learn to see those ripples more clearly, then maybe we'd find the deeper sense of purpose we all crave.

This desire to connect to our impact extends beyond our work. Maybe you're a parent feeling overwhelmed by the daily grind and believe that your efforts to drive your kids to and from practice, prepare dinner, and act as a homework helper go unnoticed. Or maybe you've been helping a friend through a difficult time by answering calls and texts at all hours, except that your friend doesn't seem to acknowledge it. Perhaps you've been putting in long hours for a project at your job, but no one seems to notice how hard you're working. You may be thinking, Does what I do every day even matter?

If you're feeling unseen or depleted, you don't have to wait for validation. You can start by paying attention to where your efforts are making a difference now. Connecting with your impact in this way will require a mental shift. You might start by reflecting on one small moment in the day where you made a difference. Take my husband, Peter. His work involves projects that take months or years to finish, which can make him feel disconnected from the results. That's one of the reasons he loves cooking. Making a meal gives him a tangible sense of gratification. The oohs and aahs from family and friends remind him that he's making a daily difference.

Keep an impact file

Even small reminders of our impact can make the most demanding jobs more manageable. That's the idea behind what I call an "impact file," a kind of personal treasure chest you can return to whenever you start to question whether your efforts matter. This collection can include thank-you notes, emails from clients, messages from your kids, photos, or birthday cards from friends— anything that reminds you of the difference you make in others' lives. Think of it as the opposite of a gratitude journal, where you gather the appreciation others have shown to you. Lauren Smith Brody, CEO of the workplace gender equality firm the Fifth Trimester, keeps what she calls "little contributions notes" on a Google document, compiling thank-you notes from clients and press reports on her government work. She even constructed a makeshift trophy wall for herself, where she hangs framed copies of press clippings. The act of framing sends a message to herself that her contributions are "real" and worthy of attention. As Lauren puts it, "The recognition of my efforts, even though I have to pull them out myself, motivate me to keep going."

That practice can be especially helpful given how easily we can lose sight of the positive ways we make a difference. Our brains are primed to focus on what goes wrong rather than what goes right. Researchers refer to this tendency as a "negativity bias." It's a survival tactic we inherited from our earliest ancestors to protect us from danger. But what once saved us from tigers now distorts how we see our days. Focusing on the negative can dim our view of the real difference we make. An impact file helps to override that bias and encourages us to make a conscious effort to notice the positive, too.

Just as Greg did with his "I'm telling" initiative, we can also use humor to make it easier, and therefore more habitual, to recognize the impact of others. My husband, Peter, has a family tradition of handing out quirky, inexpensive, slightly tacky trophies for anything remotely competitive, from axe throwing (don't ask) to our annual Trivial Pursuit showdown. Imagine taking this approach in an office setting, where saying "you matter" can feel awkward and forced. Years ago, Peter's workplace introduced some untraditional year-end awards. There was an award for someone who gave their all to a project that ultimately didn't come together. Another honored a partner's sound judgment in walking away from a tempting but too-risky investment—his plaque, celebrating his "rational exuberance"—still sits proudly on his shelf. Imagine giving a family member the "Glue Award" for the person who keeps everything and everyone together. These unexpected acknowledgments offer a playful way to let someone know what they do makes a difference.

Part of a bigger whole

One of the most powerful ways to connect with your impact is to recognize how your role, no matter how small it may seem, fits into a larger purpose. When we connect our efforts to something larger, we strengthen our sense of mattering in the world. Consider a janitor who once worked for NASA. In a well-loved story, during a 1962 visit to NASA's headquarters, President Kennedy encountered this janitor and asked what he was doing. The janitor replied, "I'm helping put a man on the moon." This janitor was right; he *was* helping to put a man on the moon. Seeing himself as part of the mission strengthened his sense of impact.

> *Do what you can, with what you have, where you are.*
>
> —Bill Widener

Crucially, when we can connect our roles with a greater impact, we don't just feel better, we also perform better. Research finds that chefs in open-kitchen restaurants, where they can see firsthand the finished dishes arriving at a diner's table, tend to cook better food. Seeing the smiles and reactions of diners allows chefs to understand how their efforts, such as slicing carrots, washing herbs, or sautéing vegetables, contribute to a satisfying meal. As a result, diners tend to report that the food is tastier. What's more, the chefs report greater satisfaction with their work. Seeing the bigger picture boosts the quality of their work and deepens their commitment to their craft—the two go hand in hand.

If you ever find yourself noticing how someone's impact is an important part of a whole, tell them. Maybe your colleague has been going above and beyond to ensure deadlines are met, or your neighbor has been organizing community cleanups that keep your local park beautiful. Take a moment to tell them how much this effort has lifted the energy of the workplace or neighborhood. At home, you might point out how your child's small act of kindness toward a friend creates a ripple effect of kindness in their friend group. Recognition is a way of saying, *I see the good in you.* In moments like this, people remember who they are and why they matter.

If it weren't for you . . .

Every year on a friend's birthday, Amelia, a real estate agent in Florida, sends her friends a note that begins, "If it weren't for you . . ." and then writes about the many ways they impact the world around them. For her cousin Mia, she wrote, "If it weren't for your humor, our family gatherings wouldn't be nearly as fun. Your outgoing personality helps to make us closer." For her colleague Daniel, she wrote, "If it weren't for you, our office wouldn't be as warm and friendly. You've been instrumental in creating this positive environment." Friends tell Amelia they often hold on to these letters as a reminder that people notice the best in them.

Amelia's letters strike at the deepest form of awareness, the feeling that our *absence* would impact others for the worse and would leave the world a little emptier. When we experience our impact, when we feel like we are irreplaceable in our circles, it can be transformative. Amelia's letters offer her friends this exact reassurance, pointing out that without them, the world would miss their kindness, wisdom, or humor.

At the end of each year, a friend of mine has a tradition I've come to think of as his personal acknowledgments page, like the section in a book where authors thank those who have helped them along the way. On New Year's Day, he sends an email to everyone who made his life better that year. This simple message of gratitude does two things: It makes each person who receives it feel valued, and it also reminds my friend of the web of support that surrounds him each day.

The Power of Social Networks: Researchers have found that our behaviors and emotional states can ripple through our social networks up to three degrees of separation. That means we influence not just our friends, but their friends, and even their friends' friends. In other words, your actions matter to people you may never meet.

Like Amelia and my friend, there are people who quote your words and remember your kindness toward them long after you've moved on. Traces of your efforts are everywhere, even if they aren't always visible. To paraphrase the words of Scottish poet Donna Ashworth: "If every single person [you have impacted] in your lifetime, were to light up on a map, it would create the most glitteringly beautiful network you could imagine. Throw in the strangers you've been kind to, the people you've made laugh, or inspired along the way. . . . You're trailing a bright pathway that you don't even know about. What a thing. *What a thing indeed.*"

Greg, too, knows the impact that a person's absence can leave on the world. A year before Greg took over as fire chief, on June 18, 2007, the Charleston Sofa Super Store was engulfed in a catastrophic fire. This fire would forever change firefighting in the region and beyond. It started on the store's loading dock, where packing materials caught on fire. Within minutes, the fire spread inside to the store's highly flammable furniture. From the outside, the blaze appeared manageable. But what the firefighters couldn't know was that the building was on the brink of collapse. As the fire intensified, firefighters from the Charleston Fire Department, the neighboring department to North Charleston, were trapped inside as the heat, poor visibility, and rapidly deteriorating conditions overwhelmed them. Tragically, nine firefighters lost their lives that day.

It was one of the deadliest firefighting tragedies in US history. Investigations into the disaster found critical failures, like inadequate hoses and poor communication. It prompted nationwide changes in training, equipment, and safety protocols. As fire chief, Greg took those painfully learned lessons and used them to create a new firehouse culture that focused on continuous training and open communication and collaboration. When Greg retired after twenty-seven years of service in January 2024, his mind returned to the Sofa Super Store fire. "Those men presented firefighters all around the country with a unique opportunity to change," Greg said, choking up and looking away. While these young men could never be replaced, Greg and his team could carry forward their legacy in how every firefighter trained and every call was answered. As he stepped out of the uniform, Greg felt an overwhelming need to honor those men once more.

There's a grassy field on the site where the Charleston Sofa Super Store once stood, with a memorial that honors those nine firefighters. Plaques have been carefully placed across the site. Each one marks the spot where a firefighter's body was found. For the people of Charleston, the memorial serves as a reminder of the danger and sacrifice their firefighters confront daily. In many ways, the memorial is also a monument of awareness and proof that these men had an impact far beyond their final moments.

About a month after his retirement, Greg drove out to visit the memorial alone. In his pocket were nine Chief Coins. One by one, Greg knelt before the plaques and placed a coin. The coins were Greg's way of saying, *I see you. You mattered.*

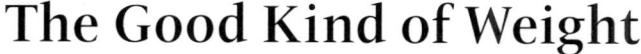

CHAPTER 2

The Good Kind of Weight

The Mattering Core

Recognition: You and your actions are valued, and your absence would be felt.

Reliance: You feel needed because others depend on you.

Importance: You feel significant because you're prioritized.

Ego Extension: You feel cared for because others are invested in your well-being.

Attunement: You feel deeply understood and meaningfully responded to.

Julie Plaut Mahoney stepped into the foyer of her childhood home and let the silence settle in around her. The faint scent of her mother's perfume now made her ache. It all felt too intimate to be in her mother's house without her there. As Julie walked through the rooms, she took in the objects left behind: her mother's reading glasses, a wooden elephant from Thailand, and a favorite throw blanket. In the kitchen, her eyes went to the empty yellow soup pot on the stove, a witness to a lifetime of family meals.

Her mother Linda's illness came as a shock. During a 2017 family trip to the Berkshires, Julie and her brother noticed Linda was limping. The next day doctors diagnosed her with stage IV glioblastoma, a fast-growing brain cancer. Linda's independence vanished overnight. The car keys were taken. She would need full-time care. Still, Linda was determined to keep working as the director of cultural affairs of Newton, Massachusetts, where she organized concerts, festivals, and public art. To help her do that and to ensure her final months felt meaningful, Julie decided to become Linda's full-time caregiver. This meant Julie would resign from her job as a volunteer manager at Newton at Home, a nonprofit that supports older adults. While Julie loved her work, she realized the most urgent need right now was closer to home. Julie's brother supported this decision and her sacrifice by contributing financially to their mother's care.

While an aide cared for her mother overnight, Julie took the day shift. Every morning, Julie drove the mile and a half to her childhood home. From nine a.m. to four p.m., Julie was her mother's driver, personal assistant, and home health aide. Linda relied on Julie to get her to meetings and maintain some semblance of the life she cherished, and Julie was comforted that she was able to honor Linda's wish to stay engaged with the world for as long as possible.

Linda worked remotely until the very end of her life, spending her final weekend raising thousands of dollars for an upcoming concert. A few days later she passed away. The grief was immediate and consuming. Not only had Julie lost her only living parent, she also lost the sense of purpose and identity that came from being relied on in such a profound way. For nineteen months,

Julie's life had revolved around her mother's care, going grocery shopping, checking medications, and making sure her mother's slippers were within reach. Now, an unsettling sense of weightlessness crept over her. The emptiness of the days and weeks ahead filled her with dread. Who was she, she wondered, if not a daily caregiver? "There was this vastness, this chasm, this gap," Julie said. "I'm not sure you know how meaningful that is to you until it is no longer there."

Meanwhile, she also faced a more practical dilemma: What would she do with all of her mother's belongings? The candy dish, the yellow pot, the china set—every object held a memory. How could she possibly decide what to keep and what to throw away? These belongings, much like Julie herself, needed a new purpose.

In her work with Newton at Home, Julie had encountered many families in similar situations. In the overwhelming days following a loss, families wondered what to do with homes full of their loved ones' belongings. Julie suggested ways to repurpose them: perhaps that old set of pots and pans could be donated to a family in the community who lost their home in a fire or to refugees who were building a life in Newton from scratch. Over time, these suggestions grew into a regular operation. Together with her friend Mindy Frankel Peckler, Julie picked up items left out for them on porches and front steps and stored them in a room in a friend's office until they could match the items with someone who could use them. Soon the program became so popular that Julie and Mindy relocated their operation to a larger room on the first floor of a church. Even after stepping down from her role at Newton at Home, Julie had continued to run the program with Mindy.

Standing in her mother's kitchen, she realized it was her turn to do the same with her mother's belongings, to give them a second life. Another thought occurred to her: What if she and Mindy expanded the project into something larger? What if, instead of working one donation at a time, they created a more efficient system that could reach more people? Starting a nonprofit, she thought, would allow them to formalize their efforts and apply for grants that would help them to grow their impact. Three months after her mother's passing, Julie and Mindy "gave birth," as Julie put it, to their nonprofit Welcome Home. Julie remembered feeling like a baby deer on shaky legs: "It was like, okay, we're really going to do this now."

On the day I visited Welcome Home, volunteers stood at a long table preparing kitchen kits, laughing, and working together like a family. It struck me how Julie transformed her personal loss into something meaningful by looking outward for new ways to be depended on again. Watching her, I wondered, What if the very thing we fear will drain us—reliance—is actually what helps to restore us?

Turn outward

We don't need to start a nonprofit to become someone others can depend on. Often, it's small gestures that can open that door. Maybe you're the kind of person who, like my friend Lisa, shares her freshly baked bread with friends, a gift we all look forward to and associate with her warmth and care. Perhaps you're the neighbor people turn to when they have a problem, such as a stuck window or a dead car battery, because you never make them feel like a burden. Through steady acts of generosity like these, we become essential to the people around us.

> **To add value = Find a need in the world +**
> **Apply your strengths**

When I asked Julie what advice she'd give to someone feeling adrift like she was after her loss, she paused, then said simply, "Stop looking at the mirror for an hour a week." That hour, she implied, could be better spent turning outward and doing something useful for someone else. What Julie was pointing out is that when we're hurting or stretched thin, the instinct is often to retreat. We might tell ourselves that we are too overwhelmed to take on anything else, or perhaps assume that we need to be fully healed or whole before others can depend on us.

That's because we often think of energy as a finite resource, like water in a glass; we fear that if we keep pouring, it will run out. But energy doesn't always work that way. Studies consistently show that helping others boosts our vitality, what researchers have termed a "helper's high." One study found that regular volunteering was linked to higher levels of energy and well-being. Another study found that those who spent time helping others reported having *more* time available in their day than those who spent time on themselves. Researchers theorized this is because helping others makes us feel more capable and more in control of our schedules. That shift to turn our lens outward can be small, like offering to walk a neighbor's dog while they recover from surgery, mentoring a younger colleague who's struggling, or cooking a double batch of dinner and bringing half to a new parent down the street. Instead of burning us out, turning outward can light us up by reminding us just how essential we are to others.

There's a growing tendency in our culture to treat responsibility to others as an inconvenience, an obligation to dodge or delegate. In trying to guard against burnout or preserve autonomy, we can begin to see every task as a threat, like one more thing to manage rather than a sign that we matter. But responsibility and obligation aren't the same thing. *Obligation* comes from the Latin *obligare*—to bind. It implies duty without choice. *Responsibility*, by contrast, comes from *respondere*—to respond. It's grounded in agency. Where obligation says "you have to," responsibility says "you can." One feels like weight, while the other feels like an invitation. When we conflate the two, we miss something essential. When no one depends on us, a sense of purposelessness can creep in. As counterintuitive as it may seem, too much freedom without meaningful responsibility can leave us feeling hollow.

The heavier the burden, the closer our lives come to the earth, the more real and truthful they become. Conversely, the absolute absence of burden causes man to be lighter than air, to soar into heights, take leave of the earth and his earthly being, and become only half real, his movements as free as they are insignificant. What then shall we choose? Weight or lightness?

—Milan Kundera

It takes a conscious shift to turn outward and see the power in choosing to care. Julie didn't collapse under the weight of her caregiving role because she didn't see it as a burden but rather as an opportunity. She understood that responsibility is like a muscle that over time builds up reliance. When we stop using it, the muscle, and our sense of mattering, atrophies.

Meet a need

Michael discovered this himself. He enjoyed his reputation as the dependable one at work, someone who could always be counted on to bring treats to the weekly meetings or to stay late when a colleague needed help. But when his company went fully remote during a merger, Michael and his colleagues packed up their things to work from home. At first, the freedom felt like a luxury: no commute, no unwelcome interruptions, and much more time to himself. For the first time in a long time, he was able to organize his day exactly the way he wanted to. But Michael lived alone. And as the novelty wore off, he began to notice something. He still chatted with colleagues on Zoom and saw friends on weekends, but there were stretches of time—days—when he realized he hadn't spoken to another person face-to-face. And though he couldn't name it at first, there was something uncomfortable about all this freedom.

After a few months of working remotely, Michael visited a pet adoption fair and was immediately drawn to a shy tabby named Blue. Michael signed the paperwork and brought Blue home. At first, Blue hid behind the back of the couch. But slowly, he started to engage: meowing at seven a.m., pawing at Michael's keyboard during meetings, and demanding playtime every evening. Blue needed attention, food, water, and care. And in meeting those small needs, Michael began to realize just how much he'd missed the feeling of being relied on. He was missing the daily signals that his presence mattered. Freedom, while appealing, had cut him off from the small, everyday ways people depended on him, a sense of reliance that gave his life structure and meaning.

Ethan discovered this, too. After graduating from college without a job lined up, Ethan spent his days sending out résumés and writing cover letters. As the weeks wore on with no job offers in sight, Ethan's morning routine started later and later in the day. Watching from the sidelines, his parents grew frustrated and then concerned. One afternoon, there was a knock at the front door. It was their neighbor, Joan. She was undergoing chemotherapy and wondered if she could pay Ethan to take her to the hospital for treatment twice a week. Ethan said yes, seeing it as a way both to make a little money and to get his parents off his back.

Ethan started driving Joan to her appointments because she

needed the help and he needed the money. But, over time, their rides became something he looked forward to. Joan told stories about her life after college. Ethan helped her in and out of the car, and as she grew weaker, that assistance became more important. When Joan mentioned feeling nauseous, Ethan made a trip to the health food store and returned with ginger tea the manager had recommended. After a few weeks, Ethan stopped accepting her money. He wanted to help Joan through her treatment because he cared about her, not because he wanted something in return. Ethan's parents noticed a change in him. He seemed more energized and purposeful about his job search. "He seemed proud again," his father told me. What looked like depression, his father said, wasn't only about not working—it was about not being needed.

> *The worst thing that could possibly happen to anybody would be to not be used for anything by anybody.*
>
> —Kurt Vonnegut

What Blue gave Michael, and what Joan gave Ethan, was the chance to add value by being relied on. Instead of weighing them down, this steady sense of reliance actually reenergized them. Needs are all around us, but recognizing them requires a shift in how we pay attention. It means noticing the everyday moments where we can step in and choosing to act. When we begin to see the world this way, everyday life becomes full of chances to make a difference. One silly example is what I like to call my "traffic BFF" ritual. When I'm having a rough day, I make it a point to let anyone I see merge ahead of me in traffic. Helping others, even in such a small way, lifts my mood. These seemingly inconsequential moments remind me that my presence can make a small difference in others' lives. Reaching out to a friend to ask how the doctor's appointment went or taking a minute to encourage a coworker before their big presentation are examples of finding and filling a need. When we begin to look for them, we see that these ordinary moments where we can fill a gap or lighten someone else's load are all around us.

Lean into your strengths

When the COVID-19 pandemic hit, the Georgia-Pacific plant in Muskogee, Oklahoma, announced its first-ever layoffs. This was a huge economic blow to the community. Local businesses also struggled, and some were forced out of business. Layoffs grew. Colton Archer, the fourth-generation owner of Archer Cleaners, a dry cleaning business, began to wonder what he could do to help his neighbors. He decided to provide free dry cleaning services to anyone who needed it, no questions asked. He knew it would be an easy way to help people look good and therefore feel good in interviews. So he and his team put posters on the doors at all four Archer Cleaners locations advertising the new program. More than twenty people took him up on the offer. One man came in to shake Colton's hand and personally thank him.

He told Colton he'd lost his apartment and was living in his car. The free dry cleaning, he said, had helped him show up with confidence to a job interview, and he got the job. Interactions like this made Colton feel that he was adding value to others' lives. Long after the pandemic ended, the posters are still up, and Colton said he has no plans to take them down.

Colton found his way to a need by first reflecting on what he was uniquely positioned to offer. As the owner of a dry cleaning business, his ability to clean and press clothes allowed him to meet a tangible need in a way that felt doable and impactful. All of us can learn from Colton's approach. What skills, resources, and strengths do you have that could help someone else? Strengths don't have to be standout skills but rather anything you enjoy and feel relatively comfortable doing, like organizing events or knowing how to create a cozy atmosphere that invites community. If you're unsure of your strengths, start by asking yourself simple questions like, "What activities make me lose track of time?" or "What do people thank me for, even casually?" Asking close friends and family what they see as your talents can also help bring them into focus.

The next step is to consider how to use those strengths to meet the needs around you. My friend's eighty-four-year-old father-in-law has always loved lawn care and landscaping and takes pride in keeping his yard neat and tidy. So, he volunteers to maintain the landscaping at his church, mows his neighbors' lawns, and in the winter snow-blows neighbors' driveways. Years after he retired as a small-business owner, this practice makes him feel relevant and useful. By matching what he loves to do with a need in his community, he found a lasting way to feel needed and stay connected.

Invite someone to help

Every Tuesday and Friday, without fail, Daniel calls his dad. He asks for advice on how to fix the leaky faucet, navigate a tricky social dynamic at work, or cook a steak in the best way. These calls are about more than getting answers. Daniel has watched his dad struggle to find his place in the world since retiring. Daniel understands, when he hears the energy return in his dad's voice, that being depended on gives his dad a renewed sense of purpose. It's moments like these that prove to his dad that he is still needed.

When we ask someone for advice, we affirm their value. Psychologists call this "the advice-giving effect"—when someone shares wisdom, they feel more appreciated and competent. "Human beings are basically wired to want to give help," social psychologist Heidi Grant explains. "It's one of the richest sources of self-esteem."

Sharing information is an easy way to fill a need, too. Take my brother-in-law Andrew, who makes a point of keeping track of birthdays and anniversaries. Every so often, a text from him will appear in our family group chat: "Don't forget, it's Erin's birthday tomorrow." His shift in focus, from keeping this knowledge to himself to sharing it with the family, allows all of us to recognize these special days and helps keep our family connected.

Others use that same instinct to fill a need for their wider communities. One woman I interviewed maintains a weekly list of free events, food pantries, and community programs, which she shares in local online groups. One of her posts helped a family find a free school supply giveaway right before the start of the school year, and another connected a neighbor with a low-cost health clinic. Her efforts show how sharing information can bridge gaps, allowing people to access the support they need and inspiring others to step in and help where they can. If you volunteer at a food bank on weekends, ask a neighbor or colleague to come along. If you're passionate about sustainability, invite your colleagues to join you in a simple challenge, like a "no-plastic week" at work. When we act as "mattering matchmakers," we become part of something bigger.

Be a matchmaker

The Repair Café, started in Amsterdam in 2009, is an excellent example of matchmaking. Instead of throwing away everyday items, like broken lamps or toasters, people bring them to the "café" and learn how to repair them, meet their neighbors, and reduce landfill waste. The concept quickly spread, with more than 2,500 Repair Cafés popping up across Europe and beyond.

In 2013, John Wackman, an environmental advocate, brought the Repair Café to New Paltz, New York. He saw how many perfectly fixable items ended up in landfills simply because people lacked the skills or tools to repair them. More than that, he saw an opportunity to invite others to help. John recruited volunteer fixers, from mechanically inclined neighbors to retired engineers, tailors, and electricians, and invited them to share their skills with the community. Beyond fixing things, John hoped to repair the connection between people in his community.

The impact was immediate. Neighbors who had never met sat side by side, learning to sew a button, rewire a lamp, or fix a treasured toy. Skilled volunteers found purpose in teaching, and those seeking help left not just with repaired items but sometimes with new relationships.

Take William, a retired handyman who struggled with not being relied upon after closing his business. At the Repair Café, he put his skills to use again. "This has given me a new purpose," he says. "It fills a hole in my retirement." Another volunteer, Michelle, told me she cared about sustainability but struggled to turn this interest into a way she could make a meaningful impact. Discovering the Repair Café has been "magical," she said. It is an outlet where she can apply her knowledge—she has degrees in environmental science and fashion—to make a difference. And she loves her interactions with others, especially watching "the joy and gratitude in the salvation of a beloved item." In a time when technology often replaces human interaction, when our disposable culture tells us that old things (and sometimes people) are obsolete, the Repair Café offers a counternarrative: Nothing and no one is disposable.

As John's story shows us, thinking locally doesn't mean ignoring global issues. Instead, it allows us to see that big problems, like climate change, have roots in individual lives, neighborhoods, and communities. For example, repairing furniture instead of discarding it keeps items out of landfills and avoids the emissions tied to manufacturing and transporting new goods. This means that even one small act, such as fixing a chair, can reduce both waste and the carbon footprint associated with replacing it. In other words, the ripples of our small actions don't stay small. They travel outward, touching lives far beyond our own.

Use pain as a compass

Sometimes pain, anxiety, or other difficult emotions can point us to areas where we or those around us need support. These feelings, while uncomfortable, can reveal opportunities to make a difference. The Netflix film *Joy*, for instance, is based on the story of Jean Purdy, a nurse reportedly suffering from endometriosis, a medical condition that left her unable to conceive but also fueled her determination to help others achieve what she could not. Her lab work and empathy offered groundbreaking contributions to in vitro fertilization (IVF), leading to the birth of Louise Brown, the world's first "test-tube baby." By the time of her death, Jean Purdy had helped bring hundreds of children into the world through IVF, an innovation that would go on to transform millions of lives and families across the globe. Purdy transformed her personal pain into a gift for millions of families.

The purpose of life is not to be happy—but to matter, to be productive, to be useful, to have it make some difference that you lived at all.

—Leo Rosten

The question "What keeps you up at night?" can channel worries into action. Maybe you're worried that your friend, a new parent, seems more isolated lately. This worry might prompt you to check in on her with a phone call or a visit. One mom in Idaho, who was sleepless over the presidential election, created an Instagram post on election day that read, "Anyone need a sitter today so you can get out and vote?" Her insomnia became a catalyst for action.

Perhaps you're kept awake by pangs of loneliness after moving to a new city. By paying attention to this loneliness, you might join a local group, volunteer, or organize a meetup. Such action transforms your own loneliness into an opportunity to help others who may feel the same. This was true for Brianna Kohn, who started a group called City Girls Who Walk after many of her friends had moved out of New York City during the pandemic. She was lonely and eager for friendship. As a personal trainer, she posted an open invitation on TikTok, inviting her followers to join her for a walk. The response was overwhelming—more than 250 women, mostly in their twenties and thirties, showed up. Since that day, City Girls Who Walk has sparked similar walking groups in cities across the US and at least one in Europe. Kohn's pangs of loneliness grew into a group that has become a source of connection and community for lonely people everywhere.

Don't assume—ask

Offering something meaningful ultimately requires us to look beyond ourselves and let others show us where support is most needed. Sometimes all it takes is asking *"What can I do to help?"* to find a genuine need. Consider Paul Feiner, who, for over thirty years, has worked as town supervisor for Greenburgh, New York, overseeing daily operations, budgeting, finances, law enforcement, planning, community relations, and the administration of local government. It's a busy job, but Paul doesn't make his constituents schedule appointments to see him. Instead, he comes to them. On top of the car he drives around town is a sign that reads "Mobile Problem Solver." Throughout the year, he rides his bike around town, stopping people on the street to ask, "Do you have any concerns?"

Some people told him they needed a pothole fixed, so Paul photographed it and uploaded the image to an app called "Fix It! Greenburgh," which funnels concerns to Public Works. One resident requested increased pedestrian safety measures, so Paul started giving out pedestrian reflectors for free. Another woman wanted a new playground for her neighborhood, so he helped make it happen. When the same woman pointed out that there was no way to safely walk kids to the new playground, Paul helped allocate funds for a sidewalk, which will be built next year.

As Paul shows so well, when we ask instead of assume, we create space for others to define what their needs actually are. This can be as straightforward as reaching out to a friend or colleague and asking, "Is there anything you could use help with right now?" Stacey, a woman I spoke with, took this approach with a friend of hers who lost her husband. When Stacey said she wanted to find a way to help, her friend said it would be nice to wake up to a text in the mornings. Waking up to an empty bed was particularly difficult. A morning text, she said, would make her feel more connected and less alone. Stacey now looks forward to this small ritual with her friend. She said, "It's such a gift when someone tells you how you can help."

For someone who prefers indirect support, it might look like, "Hey, I'm heading to Costco. What can I pick up for you?" These "need nudges" convey genuine interest in meeting people where they are, that we're not there to "fix" others but to better understand and support them. The golden rule, "Do unto others as you would have them do unto you," invites us to treat others with the same care and respect we hope to receive. But when it comes to offering meaningful support, the platinum rule, as it's commonly known, goes a step further: "Do unto others as they would want done unto themselves." This rule shifts the focus from our preferences to theirs. Instead of assuming what someone needs based on what we would appreciate, we fill a genuine need by taking the time to understand what would actually feel supportive to them.

Fostering reliance through trust

Finding a need and meeting it is the first step toward fostering reliance. But a single act, however generous, is just the beginning. The next step is to build the element of trust. Trust forms as actions are repeated over time, signaling that others can count on you. It might look like following through when you say you will and demonstrating that your care isn't fleeting. Each repeated action adds another layer to strengthen that trust. Over time, as you keep meeting needs, you begin to weave yourself into a web of mutual care, a kind of belonging where your well-being is tied to others', and theirs to yours.

Take Welcome Home, for example. What started with Julie finding and filling a need turned into genuine reliance in her community. In 2019, an anonymous donation allowed Welcome Home to move out of the church basement and into a bright warehouse just off Newton's main street. Julie, Mindy, and their team transformed it into a warm, thoughtfully curated simulation of a home goods store, filled with kitchenware, linens, and decor, including items that once belonged to Julie's mother. Referred by social workers, clients arrive to find prepacked bundles wrapped like gifts, along with the freedom to choose five free decorative items, like pillows or artwork, to make their space feel personal. It has become a place of dignity, choice, and new beginnings for families starting over after homelessness, domestic violence, or being displaced. "You see it in their faces," Julie said. "They've been through so much. But then they find something— a towel, a lamp, a blanket—and it's like the foundation of a new chapter begins to take shape."

Donors, too, feel the ripple effect. Whether it's Julie watching a man joyfully take home her mother's china or Mindy writing heartfelt thank-you notes when she receives donations, there's meaning in knowing beloved items will go on to serve someone else. In just five years, Welcome Home has become a vital community bridge, connecting those in need with those who want to help. In other words, the community has come to rely on and trust Julie and Welcome Home to help them navigate some of the darkest moments of their lives.

This same trust also allows the volunteers to rely on one another. When one volunteer lost her husband, she returned to her shift within a couple of weeks. Though still deep in grief, those familiar hours spent sorting and packing donations gave her a way to connect with others, even briefly. This woman knew she could trust Julie and the others to provide a safe, welcoming environment where her grief could simply exist without judgment.

Julie has earned that trust by keeping Welcome Home predictable and well-structured for volunteers. Every shift begins and ends exactly on time. Each person knows their role. "If a non-profit feels disorganized," Julie explained, "volunteers won't feel like their time is being used well." By establishing clear guidelines and consistent routines—like assigning volunteers to regular shifts on Monday and Wednesday mornings—she creates an environment where people know what to expect. Building routines and habits that allow others to count on you takes time and effort, but, as Julie has discovered, it's one of the most rewarding ways to make a lasting impact.

Do small things with great love

We never know when a brief moment of kindness—filling a small need—might set us on the path toward something greater. Perhaps helping a coworker with a project leads to a deep friendship, or taking time to listen to a neighbor creates a meaningful bond that lasts for decades. While most acts of kindness will remain isolated gestures, even when nothing more comes of them, they are still important. Every act of kindness, no matter how small, reflects a choice to see and value another person and creates ripples of goodness that we may never fully understand.

> **The Butterfly Effect:** A small act can have a ripple effect far beyond what we can see. In chaos theory, the butterfly effect describes how something as small as a butterfly flapping its wings can set off a chain reaction that leads to a tornado weeks later, halfway around the world. It's a poetic way of capturing this truth: Our actions—no matter how small—carry weight. A kind word, a generous gesture, a thoughtful pause to really see someone: These moments often land more deeply than we realize. In a world that can make us feel invisible or unimportant, the butterfly effect is a reminder: Your presence matters. Your impact ripples.

This idea resonates across spiritual traditions, emphasizing the often unseen power of doing good for others. We often refer to the many small ways we fill a need daily as "random acts of kindness," but many spiritual traditions see these acts as responses to a higher calling. For example, in Judaism, the concept of *tikkun olam*, or "repairing the world," calls for people to improve society through both individual and collective action, the idea that we all share in the responsibility of building a just and compassionate world. Similarly, Christianity encourages us to embody the kind of compassion that places collective well-being above our self-interest and to love our neighbor as ourself. The story of the Good Samaritan highlights how compassionate acts fulfill this higher purpose. We can also look to Hinduism's principle of *ahimsa*—nonviolence and genuine care toward all living beings—or Islam's practice of *zakat*, which emphasizes each person's responsibility to support the vulnerable. In Buddhism, the concept of *karuna* (compassion) calls people to actively alleviate suffering, seeing compassion as an essential action that dissolves boundaries between self and others. What all of these concepts have in common is the belief that each person's everyday actions reach far beyond their immediate circle in ways that are invisible and important. This kind of "existential reliance" recognizes that each one of us plays a unique and critical role in keeping the world in balance.

A few years ago, I sat on a bench in a park with tears rolling down my face after receiving a call I had been dreading for five years. My dear friend had just told me her cancer treatments were no longer working. She was transitioning to hospice. The finality of the news suddenly hit me. As I sat there and cried, a woman I'd never met approached and gently held out a bottle of water—still cold, fresh from a nearby vendor. "Do you need anything?" she asked quietly. It was a small gesture. But in that moment, it felt like the world was reminding me I wasn't alone. That simple act of care has stayed with me ever since, proof that even fleeting moments of kindness can leave an imprint.

There's a quote often attributed to Mother Teresa: "Not all of us can do great things. But we can do small things with great love." I've come to hold that quote close as a kind of guidance. We don't always get to fix the pain, change the outcome, or rewrite the story. But we can all be that extended hand. I've come to believe that this reliance is the counterweight to the hollow parts of modern life. When we're not needed, when no one relies on us, our lives can feel disconcertingly weightless. That's the ache Julie described after her mother passed away. What helped her climb out of that fog, what grounded her again, was the good weight of meaningful responsibility.

When I asked Julie what gave her the strength to push through her lowest moments, she pointed to her mother's influence. "She always had a purpose, whether through paid or volunteer work," she said. Julie told me her mother modeled this middle ground of being both there for the family and engaged with the world. At Welcome Home, Julie has found her way to carry on that legacy. "If you're in a hole, feeling like you don't matter, go somewhere you're needed, where you're relied on, where people depend on you," Julie said. "You have a responsibility to make yourself useful again."

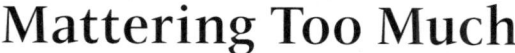

CHAPTER 3

Mattering Too Much

The Mattering Core

Recognition: You and your actions are valued, and your absence would be felt.

Reliance: You feel needed because others depend on you.

Importance: You feel significant because you're prioritized.

Ego Extension: You feel cared for because others are invested in your well-being.

Attunement: You feel deeply understood and meaningfully responded to.

Danna Thomas stood in the middle of her classroom and took it all in: The turquoise walls and fluffy clouds that she and a friend had painted to brighten up the room. A colorful story-time rug. An interactive word board, where her students could practice sight words and build vocabulary. A reading nook. On the wall was a giant "Let's Go Fly a Kite" sign, a nod to the song from *Mary Poppins*, which would be the classroom's theme for the year. When Danna greeted her kindergarten students the next day, she'd be dressed up as Mary Poppins herself—and, as Mary Poppins did for the Banks children, she hoped to infuse their first days in school with wonder. She could hardly wait.

Danna started her teaching career with Teach for America in the Baltimore public school district. Her students faced steep challenges: poverty, food insecurity, and neighborhoods that were unsafe even during the day. These challenges only fueled Danna's determination. She knew firsthand how much a dedicated teacher could transform a child's trajectory, as her teachers had done for her when she was struggling with anxiety as a young student. And she was excited to be teaching kindergartners—students at the very beginning of their learning journeys.

However, a few months into the school year, the demands of teaching quickly piled up in ways Danna hadn't anticipated. Her classroom door was always open—literally and figuratively—and she almost always stayed late to set up the next day's activities or sit and listen to a colleague or a parent who needed her. When she took a sick day, she had to search a list of substitute teachers at six a.m. to find someone who could cover at the last moment. But, more often than not, other teachers in the building would have to cover, she told me, resulting in increased tension among the staff. Even scheduling a routine dentist appointment required her to coordinate her absence months in advance. The sheer number of students in her classroom—thirty-nine—meant that taking attendance, distributing supplies, and transitioning between activities took longer than expected, often cutting into valuable instruction time. Noise levels could quickly spiral. With so many children to care for, it sometimes felt impossible to make sure each child felt supported. There just wasn't enough of her to go around. Still, Danna tried to take it all in stride. Teaching was not just a job but a calling.

Danna subsisted on a diet of caffeine and sugar to get through her hectic days. Technically, she was entitled to a bathroom break every three hours, but most days, it didn't happen. The untreated UTIs she developed became so painful she once spent six hours teaching while holding back tears, only to wait in urgent care after school to see a doctor.

Despite these challenges, Danna was determined to appear composed around more experienced educators she really admired, like third-grade teacher Amanda, whose no-nonsense demeanor intimidated her a bit, and fellow kindergarten teacher Heather, whose gentleness seemed to cast a kind of spell on her students. *They have it all figured out, while I'm barely holding on*, Danna thought. Determined to match their confidence, she threw herself into the job even harder. "Martyrdom was normalized," she later reflected. "Staying late, working sick, and burning out were badges of honor."

One afternoon, as the bell signaled the last class of the day, Danna was caught in the middle of the end-of-day chaos. Her students were darting in every direction: One student tugged at her sleeves, another student had wet themselves, and a third began crying because they had lost their favorite eraser. Danna's arms were full of books she was trying to organize. She tried to raise her voice above the noise, but her students didn't listen. She felt herself unraveling. When the school day ended, she walked into Heather's classroom and burst into tears.

"I'm failing here," Danna cried. "I don't know how to do this." It was the first time she had allowed her vulnerability to show.

"Danna, you're not failing," Heather said gently. "You're human.

This isn't about you not being good enough. This is about the system. We're not getting the support we need."

Heather's words caught Danna off guard. For the first time, someone had named the tension she felt but couldn't articulate: The lack of resources and the endless demands were making her feel that her needs were unimportant.

To help cope with the stress at work, Danna started seeing a therapist, who nudged her to carve out time each day to take lunch with colleagues and to treat her job "like any other grown-up profession." Danna thought immediately of Amanda and Heather. When she tentatively suggested getting together for lunch, she half expected the idea to be brushed aside because everyone was so busy. Instead, Amanda and Heather agreed without hesitation.

That first lunch with Amanda and Heather felt like a revelation. They met outside, unpacking homemade salads and sandwiches, and agreed to one ground rule: No work talk. Instead, Amanda talked about how difficult it was to juggle the demands of work with parenting. Danna opened up about her recent breakup with a long-term boyfriend. Through this conversation, Danna realized that her colleagues cared about her beyond her role as a teacher. No one checked emails or watches or looked like they were rushed to return to work. It made Danna feel, for the first time in a long time, that she was important, too.

Always last

While feeling relied on is a grounding force, reminding us of the value we add, true mattering requires a balance between adding value to others and feeling valued ourselves, notes psychologist Isaac Prilleltensky. When the balance goes off-kilter, when the responsibilities pile up without enough support beneath them, that same sense of being relied on can begin to crush us. Often, it's the piling on that tilts us to overwhelm—the work deadlines being moved up, another friend in crisis, and the kids home sick again. Or maybe there's a new diagnosis in the family, and suddenly you're in charge of all the doctor visits, medication schedules, rehab therapy, and nighttime needs. Maybe you're spearheading a work project, and you haven't slept in weeks. Or maybe, like Danna, you're in charge of thirty-nine young students who so desperately need your attention you can't possibly take a bathroom break. At first, the demands feel meaningful. They remind us that we are depended on, that we matter. But over time, the weight of them can leave us feeling depleted. We begin to live a paradox, that we are central to everyone else's needs while our own needs are constantly sidelined.

> **High demands + Low support = Overwhelm**

But this isn't true mattering. It's a distorted kind of mattering, one that lacks the critical ingredient of *importance.* Mattering researcher Gordon Flett calls importance the feeling of being significant or valued. What I've learned from talking to people is that the term points to a specific experience; that is, to feel important is to feel that you are *prioritized* by others in some way.

It is the affirmation that others put us first when it counts, a signal that we aren't just seen or needed but chosen over other obligations.

If recognition is the foundation of mattering, assuring us that others notice our presence and impact, then importance builds on this foundation by transforming that awareness into action. Imagine a colleague who is visibly stressed at work. Her team notices, but if no one offers to stop what they're doing to help lighten her workload, she remains "seen" but not prioritized. Or picture a partner who realizes their significant other is exhausted from middle-of-the-night feedings. They might acknowledge it verbally—"You look exhausted." But if they continue their day without offering support, the acknowledgment can feel like nothing more than an observation.

Being prioritized tells us that others care enough to act on what they see; that is, they notice it and they adjust to support us. Think about how it touches you when your partner leaves a work meeting to join you at a doctor's appointment or when a friend rearranges her plans to be by your side during a particularly difficult time. These actions indicate that someone considers you significant enough to take precedence over everything else, at least right now. These adjusting acts are a powerful way of saying, "You're *more important than* . . . [the day's plans, the project schedule, other friends]." The choice costs something, be it time, convenience, or opportunity, and that cost becomes evidence of our importance.

Without feeling a sense of importance, we can lose steam and burn out. This feeling doesn't necessarily arrive dramatically, but rather it can creep in slowly, draining the person who has spent too long giving without receiving in return. Caregivers— teachers, medical professionals, and parents—are especially vulnerable to mattering too much and feeling important too little. The feeling can be the same even when we don't have a million responsibilities but others in our lives do, and we consistently feel last on their list. Maybe you keep trying to schedule time with a friend, only to have to reschedule and then reschedule again. Maybe you told your boss you'd like to meet, but her overload of deadlines and clients means she never puts you on the calendar. You try to shake it off, but you feel like an afterthought. I remember when, before I had my kids, my close friend Lee had two little ones. We'd be deep in a phone conversation when suddenly she'd say, "JB, gotta go," and hang up because one of her kids needed her. The phone line would just go dead. It stung.

One woman I interviewed told me that it wasn't loneliness she struggled with as a single, childless woman in her forties. She had a wide circle of friends and great colleagues. It was being "no one's number one," never the person someone else prioritized and arranged their life around.

The pay-to-play village

Part of the reason so many people feel a lack of importance today is because the world around them has fundamentally changed. Take parenting. Being a parent has always been demanding, but two major cultural shifts have intensified the pressure. First, the standards of parenting have skyrocketed. What once defined a "good parent"—keeping kids safe, fed, and loved—has now become an impossible ideal. Today's parents are expected to anticipate every need, optimize every moment, and be emotionally available twenty-four seven. According to Pew Research, over the past fifty years, the time that fathers spend on childcare has almost tripled, while mothers' time has increased 57 percent, even as 71 percent are now working outside the home. While the expectations have multiplied, the hours in the day have not. On top of that, the village that once surrounded and supported caregivers has, for many, disappeared. We've become more self-reliant as a culture, and that self-reliance has a cost, with the burden falling hardest on caregivers, who are now expected to be their own one-family villages. They're managing the mental, emotional, and physical load with little structural support. Affordable childcare, paid family leave, and flexible work policies remain out of reach for many.

Samantha, a mom of two young children, told me, "When a system depends on you to care for everyone else but doesn't care for you, the work feels important but you don't." Adding insult to injury, she said that the village still exists, but now, more often than not, you have to pay to access it. Many of the supports she remembers from her childhood that once came freely from a connected community have shifted into transactions. For example, childcare has always been necessary, but what used to be shared among friends or trusted neighbors has turned into formal and pricey arrangements with day cares and sitters. The kind of parenting wisdom once passed around at the playground or at an aunt's kitchen table now comes from paid parent coaches or online courses. Even simple acts of connection, like a friend checking in or offering a listening ear, have been supplanted by paid wellness groups or digital memberships promising support. This pay-to-play village building is financially unattainable for many.

As a result, we have a generation of parents who must over-function while feeling undersupported, believing that no matter how much they give, it's never enough. This overwhelm is something we often neglect in the conversation about youth mental health—that the adults in their lives are suffering, too, and at the same rates, according to data at Harvard's Making Caring Common. Without proper support, the foundation will crack under the pressure. Young people are feeling this growing unsteadiness, with nearly 40 percent saying they're worried about the mental health of at least one parent.

> **Caregiver Overwhelm:** In a public health advisory, 41 percent of US parents reported that they are so stressed most days they can't function, and 48 percent say their stress is completely overwhelming compared with other adults.

It's not just parents who are lacking the village—or rather, whose village now exists behind a paywall. It's the elderly widow who must hire someone on Taskrabbit to fix her fallen gutter, something that once might have been done by a family member swinging by after work or a neighbor who noticed. With every kind of help imaginable now available for a fee, we've grown used to outsourcing care. And in doing so, we've come to expect that others should do the same. We've normalized it. A friend told me that when her mother asks her for a ride to the airport, a relatively short drive from her house, her first instinct is to think, *This is what Uber is for.* But she has to check herself, she says, because what she realized her mother is asking for isn't just the ride—it's the connection and a few minutes to be together amid their busy schedules, the feeling that she is worth the thirty-minute inconvenience.

When we do choose to show up, especially when it costs us something, those acts carry even more meaning. Giving a ride to the airport or fixing a neighbor's gutter are signals that say, *You are worth my time and effort.* In a world where almost everything can be outsourced, the things we choose *not* to outsource stand out. They become evidence of importance. The inconvenience is part of the gift. It's what transforms a task into a message that says, *You're a priority to me.*

Important but invisible

The tension of being central yet not a priority echoes across many demanding roles. That's what drew me to Simone Gorrindo, a writer and military spouse. I wanted to understand what it's like to occupy an important role that is often overlooked in our society. How did Simone navigate the paradox of what she described as "essential yet invisible"?

In 2012, Simone's husband joined the US Army, and they relocated from New York to Fort Benning, Georgia. In New York, Simone had a fulfilling editorial job and friends. After the move, she says her identity narrowed to a single label: army wife. Her husband's decision to join a special operations unit meant grueling training, dangerous missions, and frequent deployments. Simone quickly faced a truth that would reverberate over the next decade, through two pregnancies, a global pandemic, and multiple deployments: that her needs were secondary, even last, in a system that always put the mission first. "We are a fundamental kind of invisible presence," Simone said of military spouses. "But we don't get a lot of airtime because our job is to be silent."

Simone endured the dissonance she said many military spouses face, that their sacrifices are central to the success of their partner's career and to our country's safety, yet those sacrifices are often rendered invisible. Whether it's pausing their own professional careers, uprooting their lives repeatedly, or maintaining stability for their families, Simone said, spouses become the silent scaffolding holding everything together. She remembers messages from unit commanders to spouses about how critical their support for their soldiers was, that they couldn't do this without them. If ever Simone felt resentful, she felt she couldn't, and shouldn't, express her emotions. Compared to the sacrifice her spouse was making, her sacrifices were unworthy of attention.

The imbalance of not being a priority is especially difficult because it is often wrapped in conflicting messaging. You know you are important, and society may even tell you that you are important—*Parents! You are the emotional backbone of families!*— but your experience is that you are last on everyone's list. In

Danna's case, everyone in her life said teachers were important, but the lack of resources and the endless demands made her feel anything but. The dissonance can be complicated by what is sometimes called the "passion tax," which is the unwritten expectation that those in certain roles should sacrifice their personal time, needs, or well-being because they love or feel passionate about their work. *You love your country, don't you? You chose to become a teacher, right?* We often carry this expectation ourselves, feeling guilty for wanting a break or to have our needs met.

Others might be tempted, like Danna, to believe their own personal failings are the reason for their fatigue and resentment. What if I organized my time better? Tried harder? Our culture reinforces this inward focus by insisting that the answer to our exhaustion lies in personal optimization or self-care. But these solutions are like Band-Aids on a wound that needs stitches. So how can we course correct?

Mattering to yourself

When we feel last on everyone's list, it's easy to start seeing ourselves that way, too. We stop asking for help, defer our needs, and convince ourselves that self-sacrifice is noble. But mattering isn't only about how others treat us; it's also about how we treat ourselves. The path back to a sense of worth begins with asking, "Am I insisting on my own importance?"

No matter how busy Danna, Amanda, and Heather were, their shared lunches became a regular occurrence. If the weather was nice, they met outside. On cold or rainy days, they met in one of their classrooms. They treated this time together like "a sacred container," as Danna put it, a space where they could be open with one another. If one was quiet or seemed preoccupied, the other two would urge her to speak first. Once, Danna opened up about crying in her car each morning before school. Instead of dismissing her, Amanda and Heather listened without judgment. You don't have to hold it in with us, they assured her. We've been there, too.

This practice of prioritizing one another for a few minutes each day gradually shifted how Danna thought about herself. In subtle yet significant ways, she relinquished her role as the martyr. She closed her classroom door to protect her planning time, set limits on how long she spent working after school, and was intentional about her meals and eating healthier. On Fridays, Danna allowed herself the simple pleasure of stepping off campus for an iced coffee. "That experience of being a priority for someone else helped me begin to understand how important it was for *me* to prioritize myself, too," she told me.

One person who taught me about treating myself like a priority is my mother-in-law, who made a conscious effort to prioritize herself in small ways. For example, she lived in a one-hundred-year-old house with closets that would be considered modest by today's standards. Yet she transformed them into something special, just for her eyes. In her bedroom closet, she hung elegant wallpaper and added brass hooks to hold scarves or purses. Shelves were adorned with decorative boxes. Even the large basement closet that held her washer and dryer was beautifully wallpapered and had a small chandelier. Opening those closets felt like stepping into a private shrine to self-respect and delight. Over the course of her life, she had come to embrace a profound truth: If we don't prioritize ourselves, no one else will. The simple act of decorating her private spaces was a bold affirmation of her importance, an everyday reminder that her joy mattered, too.

When *we* feel last on everyone's list, it can be helpful to stop what we're doing and recalibrate our view of ourselves. Am I insisting on my own importance? Am I treating myself like a priority? To even ask these questions may seem, at first, like a selfish act. Won't I let down the people counting on me? Won't I fall behind on everything I need to do? But prioritizing yourself isn't about neglecting others. It allows you to have the capacity to continue serving them and yourself.

> *Self-care* is *other-focused. It's about having more and better to give to the people and things you care about.*
>
> —Educator Alexis Shepard

By treating yourself as a priority, you also create space for the relationships in your life to become more authentic. When you tell your kids, "Mom's going to the gym because taking care of my body helps me take care of you," they come to see their mom as a person with her own needs, desires, and limits. When you tell your students, "I'm taking a personal day to recharge," they learn that even adults are growing and navigating challenges. This practice goes deeper than self-care. It is about making choices that say, *My needs matter, too.* It's about drawing a boundary, taking up space, and making time for something that restores you, not as an afterthought, but as a first step. It's easy to care for yourself when everything else is handled. It's harder, and more radical, to do it when you are most needed. But that's what prioritizing yourself really is. It's a declaration of worth and a refusal to always put yourself last.

Emily, a mother in the Pacific Northwest with two small children and a full-time job, found her way back to mattering to herself through a daily walk. Regardless of the weather conditions, be it rain, snow, or subfreezing temperatures, or the tasks on her extensive household to-do list, everyone in her family understands that it is an uncompromising commitment. It isn't about the exercise; it's about insisting on one uninterrupted hour each day to come back to herself so she can continue to be there for her family, grounded and restored. In a media interview, a UK psychotherapist described a similar experience. She spoke about the guilt she felt over how desperately she relied on her daily walk to cope with the overwhelm of parenting. At one point, she confessed to her therapist, "It's as if my parenting depends on me going for a walk." Her therapist responded gently, "Yeah, because it does." *Because it does.* Whatever your "thing" is, whatever act of radical self-prioritization allows you to keep showing up for the people who rely on you—do it. *Because it does.*

Prioritize each other

Treating ourselves like a priority will only take us so far. We need people in our lives who remind us of our importance by treating us like a priority, too. As her lunches with Amanda and Heather continued, Danna grew more comfortable revealing more of her true self to her colleagues and students. On days when she was struggling with something in the classroom, she asked for help instead of pushing through. Gradually, Danna's openness to sharing herself transformed her interactions with other staff members. She began to allow others to treat her as important, too. When the custodian noticed Danna wasn't taking enough bathroom breaks, he'd wheel his mop bucket down the hall and gently say, "Go. I've got the kids." And in turn, Danna invited new teachers, particularly those who looked like they were struggling, into her lunches with Amanda and Heather.

When we make each other a priority, we create the trust and space needed to show up as our real selves and know that we are worthy of support. This is how we neutralize the dissonance in our culture. By that I'm not saying that we necessarily make the weight of overreliance less heavy. Instead, we make each other stronger and more capable of carrying the load.

I have always felt that a human being could only be saved by another human being. I am aware that we do not save each other very often. But I am also aware that we save each other some of the time.

—James Baldwin

It was through this kind of deep friendship that army wife Simone Gorrindo also felt her mattering restored. At first, jobless and without a driver's license to navigate her new city, Simone said she struggled during her husband's deployments and trainings. She felt a stark difference between herself and the other army wives. She was older, politically liberal, and childless for several years. But soon she came to experience how the spouses thought of one another, and even her, as an unnegotiable priority. A fellow wife needed help carrying a heavy rug into the house? You pushed the work deadline. A fellow wife was stranded on the side of the road in ninety-five-degree heat? You left the book club early, showed up with cold water, and waited with her for the tow truck. No matter what, no matter the inconvenience, you answered the call.

Then Simone became pregnant. One night, struggling with crippling anxiety during one of her husband's deployments, she texted another wife whose husband was also deployed. The woman invited Simone to stay the night to ease her anxiety. One night turned into several months, and Simone essentially moved in. "I felt like I was being shown the ocean for the first time," she recalled. "I didn't know that kind of kindness existed in the world." It wasn't just the generosity—it was the feeling that she was worth accommodating, worth rearranging life for. What Simone had once felt were tenuous army relationships had transformed, through intentional prioritization, into deep, meaningful bonds.

Build deeper relationships

Prioritizing one another doesn't require opening your home. It also doesn't have to require tons of time together, as I found out when researching caregiver resilience for my book *Never Enough*. Clinical psychologist and researcher Suniya Luthar found that deliberately setting aside small chunks of time for honest, meaningful connection can profoundly reduce stress and burnout, even when our daily demands of parenting, caregiving, or work remain unchanged. In her research, Luthar created a twelve-week intervention program called Authentic Connections Groups, in which working professionals who were also mothers met for one hour per week to support one another.

To Luthar, authentic relationships mean a dynamic where both people are willing to be vulnerable with one another and to ask for support. She tested the program with busy medical professionals at the Mayo Clinic and discovered that even in this highly stressed population, carving out just that one hour per week to connect with the other women improved mental well-being and reduced levels of cortisol—the stress hormone—among the participants. One participant said how surprised she was to learn how you can create real connections in such a short time. Similar results were found with male educators who carved out this same hour of time each week. Another study found these authentic relationships can be fostered virtually as well.

Luthar's research proves that the key to these deeper, "real" connections lies not in the quantity of time spent together but in the deliberate intention to prioritize one another. Unlike relationships built on constant availability, these groups focus on creating a consistent, structured space to foster trust. The distinction reminds us that our most authentic relationships grow not necessarily from dropping everything for others all the time but by being purposeful and regularly committed to them.

Caregivers are often told to "put our oxygen mask on first." But what this research suggests is something deeper: Friends *are* the oxygen. We need people in our lives who we can open up to, who know us well enough so they can see when we are struggling for air, and who will reach over and put that oxygen mask on for us. That's a very different level of support than the one we normalize in our busy, self-reliant culture today. But I've come to think of it this way: when I don't reach out for help, not only do I deny myself the support I need—I also deny my friend the chance of being a helper, to feel trusted and relied on, to know how much they matter to me. So the next time you hesitate, I hope you'll remember that asking for help isn't weak. It is actually an act of generosity.

Feeling like a priority, even just one hour a week, is essential to keeping our mattering in balance, allowing us to add value because we also feel valued. The relationships that make us feel this way require maintenance. Think of the friend who sets a recurring monthly coffee date, the sibling who plans an annual weekend getaway, or the coworker who regularly checks in with a quick text to see how you're *really* doing—these moments don't happen by accident. They result from putting others on the calendar and protecting that time. For a spouse, this might mean setting aside one evening a week for an uninterrupted dinner or a walk together, free of distractions like phones or work. Or it might look like scheduling a weekly reminder to check in on a friend. Scheduling time signals, *I care enough about you to commit to you.*

Fight the friendship recession

Former US Surgeon General Vivek Murthy has spoken openly about combating loneliness by setting aside intentional time with friends. One of his solutions was inspired by *moai* groups originating in Okinawa, Japan—small, lifelong, intentional social circles formed to provide support and community. Murthy and his friends decided to create their own version of a moai, committing to in-depth monthly calls and more frequent text check-ins. In these calls, they discuss important topics, like the challenges of maintaining close relationships amid busy schedules and more profound questions of purpose and meaning in life. The formality of the group and the act of showing up repeatedly and reliably cement the sense that this group is a priority. Murthy was quoted in *The Washington Post* as saying this moai "has been an extraordinary force in my life that has helped ground me, has helped me feel connected, and is also helping me make critical decisions in my life about work and family."

Today, men are facing what researchers have called a "friendship recession," with 15 percent reporting that they have no close friends, a number that climbs to 20 percent if the man is single. In my interviews, the same powerful antidote emerged for men as it did for women: making time for one another with intention and consistency. I found it takes just takes one person to initiate that steady practice.

When Abraham Walker moved from a close-knit community in New Orleans to a more private suburb in Virginia, he traded the daily greetings from neighbors for a community that was less openly friendly. Sitting at his son's Little League practice, Abraham looked around at the rows of parents glued to their phones and asked himself, "Why are we all here, side by side, and yet alone?" When others said they were there to "support" their kids, Abraham couldn't shake the feeling that many simply didn't have anywhere else to go.

So Abraham pushed against the grain. He began modestly. He tried to start a book club by posting on the social networking app Nextdoor. No one came. Undeterred, he set himself an even bolder challenge: thirty coffees with thirty neighbors in thirty days. It worked. Inspired by that success, Abraham launched a dads' group on Nextdoor—a space for dads of all ages, including those with grown children. His first post drew more than two hundred responses. He set up the meetups like high school field trips, where they would first try something fun, like axe throwing, and then gather at a casual restaurant to talk. What started as a monthly event quickly turned into a weekly Friday breakfast at seven a.m. One man began attending six months before his child was born, coming for the kind of guidance he never got growing up. The group also includes dads in their seventies, proving you never stop needing community or advice. For Abraham and the others, this group has become a lifeline. "Now there's this routine to my life that just brings so much peace," he said, because he knows these men will be there for him week after week.

Mattering

*Being able to feel safe with other people is proba-
bly the single most important aspect of mental
health; safe connections are fundamental to meaningful and satisfying lives.*

—Bessel van der Kolk

Over two thousand miles away from Virginia, in a Boise, Idaho, cul-de-sac, another group of men gathers one Wednesday a month around a portable firepit with no agenda and no expectations, just lawn chairs, casual drinks, and conversation. The monthly meetup was started by a neighborhood dad who, after witnessing many of his neighbors become fathers, thought back to how he struggled with loneliness and isolation as a new parent. What he really needed—then and now—was support and community, and also just a time to be himself, not a husband or a father. His wife had this community and intentional time. She was part of an active neighborhood book club, a women-only gathering that took place once a month. Why not use that time as an excuse for the husbands to get together? Over the course of the evening, men drift in and out. Some stay for a quick chat before heading home to their families, while others linger, decompressing and swapping stories. This casual once-a-month hangout is a reminder that their need for friendship and community matters, too.

Just as children need a sturdy adult in their lives to thrive, sturdy adults need sturdy adults to lean on, too, to remain sturdy. It's so easy for the busyness of life to blur our priorities and push our friendships to the margins. But setting a recurring date, like a standing lunch or phone call, and making it a rule for yourself that you don't cancel, is an act of resistance. It's how we practice prioritizing ourselves and safeguarding our own well-being and support systems, both for ourselves and also for those relying on us. Over time, these standing moments serve as anchors, reminding us that we, too, are important and worthy of care.

Being intentional and consistent about spending time together creates the conditions for deeper conversations, the kind that strengthen trust and connection. For Danna, that meant setting the "no work talk" rule during her lunches with Amanda and Heather, allowing them to connect on a more personal level. For Abraham, this meant setting a routine he and others could rely on. For Dr. Murthy, it meant being clear about the group's purpose. In other words, we might not be outright saying, "I want to be authentic with you" or "I want to go deeper," but the structure itself sends the signal. By creating the conditions for authenticity, we make it easier for those more meaningful conversations to unfold.

Take turns

Our relationships are dynamic, and our life circumstances are ever-changing, and so to be prioritized is to feel that, because we value each other, we take turns putting each other first. When necessary, we adjust our needs, schedules, and desires for each other's benefit, just as Simone and her fellow army wives do. A few years after my friend Lee's children had left the house, the roles became reversed. Her children were grown, and I was the one with young children in the background of our calls. Now she was the one kindly tolerating my constant interruptions as I juggled snack requests. When my kids called out to me, she'd say, "JB, do you need to go?" without a hint of impatience. I understood then, as I hadn't understood before, that to be prioritized isn't to be someone's number one all the time. It's more fluid than that, more give-and-take. Sometimes, it's my turn to come first. Sometimes, it's yours.

> **Taking Turns:** Ruth Bader Ginsburg often credited her husband, Marty, for prioritizing her career and spoke often about how they both knew when to step back to allow the other to thrive. Ginsburg shared an anecdote about a call from her son's school regarding his mischievous behavior. She told the principal, "This child has two parents. Please alternate calls. It's his father's turn."

Perhaps being someone's number one isn't the only, or even the best, way of measuring that we matter. In an essay published in the online magazine *Midlife Boulevard,* a divorced empty-nester reflected, "I may not be the number one, but I'm pretty sure I'm ranked in the top ten, maybe even the top five, in many of my loved ones' lives." Her story reminds us that while we all long to feel singularly important, sometimes what matters more is being held in many hearts, in many ways. Top five, top ten— those spots count, too.

In the big picture of mattering, taking turns when it comes to feeling important is a critical counterbalance to being too overly relied upon. When we are prioritized, we are assured that others care about our needs, too. During the week between Christmas and New Year's, Welcome Home traditionally closes its doors for a break. One year, a few volunteers offered to stay open. They felt so invested in the work and the families they served that they found it difficult to step away, even briefly. But Julie and Mindy knew the value of shutting down to reset. "Despite the generous and heartfelt impulse, we closed so we could all pause and rest," Julie told me. "The goal is to keep doing this, not to give to the point of depletion." For the volunteers, the weight of reliance was balanced by the knowledge that their well-being was a priority, too. Through gestures like Julie's, importance proves that we have value beyond what we do or what we can provide.

Think about who might "need a turn" in your life. Is there someone who could benefit from a moment of attention, whose needs and contributions haven't been prioritized in a while? For Simone, her husband's turn has lasted longer than expected—it's been thirteen years and counting. But at this point in his army career, her husband is deliberately making decisions that prioritize Simone, like transitioning to a unit with a slower pace and making efforts to keep his family in Washington, where they currently live. "Nothing is guaranteed—the army could up and decide to send us to Kansas next month," she said. "But he is prioritizing his family in ways he couldn't when he was just starting out."

Even before he began this transition, Simone's husband gave her a turn in a significant way by supporting her publication of

Mattering

The Wives, a memoir about their life together and her role as an army wife. A private person by nature, Simone's husband nevertheless read multiple drafts and spent hours talking about the book with her at the kitchen table. He couldn't control his deployments or their effect on Simone. That was the nature of military life. But when it came to Simone's writing and career, he did everything he could to put her in the spotlight. For Simone, his support made her feel important by making it clear that her voice and her story mattered, too.

It's in the details

Making the people we care about feel like they're a priority doesn't have to require a big lift. Consider my mother, who consistently communicates others' importance through small, deliberate actions. She understands that mattering lies in the details. For example, she doesn't just remember that my daughter Caroline loves pasta. She remembers her favorite shape (rigatoni) and how she likes it cooked (al dente). When my son James's favorite sports team wins a game, she sends a congratulatory text. When there's a sale on the sweatshirts my son William likes, she asks if he needs any more. My mother collects these little details and preferences like treasures and then makes a point to circle back to them to show people they're a priority in her mind.

My sister Natalie is the same way. James, my youngest, spends so much time at their house during the summer, playing with his cousins, that Natalie and my brother-in-law Pete make him feel

84

at home in countless ways, such as keeping his favorite ice cream flavor in the freezer or including him in their family text chain. This kind of attentiveness to the people in our lives tells them, without words, how much they're cherished.

Making someone feel like a priority sometimes takes little more than putting a momentary spotlight on them. One way we do this in our family is with a quick, thirty-second ritual. Just about every morning, we walk each other to the door. It was my kids who started it. "Come walk me to the door"—a last little moment of connection before stepping out into the world. On the way to the door, we might chat about the day ahead. Or, if it's early and we're groggy, we don't feel pressured to say much more than "I love you." This simple routine sends the message that no matter how busy life gets, you are important. Putting down your phone when someone talks about their day, pausing the housework to help your child search for a lost toy, or stopping dinner prep to sit and listen as your partner shares about their stressful day shows the people in our lives that they are a priority.

Mattering is reinforced in those small moments. At a national conference, I once watched a teacher receive an award. The award itself was lovely, but it was the other present that visibly moved him. The presenter handed him a giant jar of his favorite afternoon treat: M&M's. His colleagues had noticed and remembered. That jar of candy said what the plaque couldn't: *You're uniquely known. Your preferences are worth remembering. You matter.* It's so easy to overlook these small gestures. But when someone pays attention to the details of our lives, like the snack we reach for or the way we like our pasta, it reminds us that we hold an important place in another person's mind. That sweet gesture from his colleagues made it clear that *he*—not just his work—was important.

Protect limits

One of the most striking lessons I learned reporting for *Never Enough* was the power of protecting limits. In a culture that sometimes treats teens like performance machines, our children can begin to feel important only for their output. But rather than continuing to push them, one way parents can make them feel important is by safeguarding their time, energy, and health. For example, we might tell our kids they don't need to pile on more AP classes or fill every spare hour with extracurriculars. Maybe we encourage them to use the summer to recharge rather than take classes. Maybe we suggest they take the weekend to rest or socialize instead of study. When we enforce these boundaries for them, we signal, *You are more important than your accomplishments.*

It's a lesson I've made conscious efforts to apply both in my parenting and in other relationships. Respecting the time and energy of others, ensuring that our demands don't push them past their limits, is a way of recognizing their finite capacity and importance. When I paid a visit to Welcome Home, I saw Julie Mahoney set clear guidelines for volunteers about their time. When one of our interviews ran up against the end of a scheduled volunteer shift, Julie stopped our conversation to ask the volunteers if they were comfortable staying an additional thirty minutes, making it clear that their time and well-being were more important than a journalist's questions. At first, I was caught off guard. It's not often that someone pauses an interview to prioritize others' time over the conversation we're having. At that moment, I wasn't thinking about importance. I was just observing, intrigued. It wasn't until later, when I was playing the scene over in my head, that I realized exactly what Julie had done. It was subtle, but the message was clear: you and your time are a priority here.

Sometimes, especially in moments of strain, the best way to protect the limits of someone in our life is to provide an emergency exit. Hospitals often use codes to signal the need for urgent attention, such as "Code Red" for fire or "Code Blue" for medical emergencies. More recently, "Code Lavender," a kind of psychological first aid, was introduced in certain healthcare settings to address the emotional and psychological needs of patients, their families, or staff members who require extra support. Later in her career, at a different school, Danna and her colleagues adopted this language for teachers facing overwhelming days. When a colleague struggled with escalating behavior issues in her classroom, she would call a "Code Lavender" to temporarily redistribute her students to other classrooms, giving her a much-needed break. The system was both practical and symbolic, sending a signal that caring for students didn't have to come at the expense of teachers' own mental health.

At other times, it might be necessary to honor our limits by removing some of the burden from our own shoulders. Not long ago, I realized I had a problem many of us share. I couldn't stop saying yes. Yes to the bake sale. Yes to the endless meetings. Yes to projects that weren't priorities but somehow landed on my plate anyway. I often felt like a pinball—someone pulled the spring back, and I was flung toward their targets and goals. While I knew something had to change, I feared disappointing people or looking like a slacker.

That's when I stumbled upon the concept of personal policies, as in simple, intentional rules meant to guide your daily decisions and actions. A personal policy might be as straightforward as "I don't answer emails after seven p.m.," or "I always take a walk during my lunch break." In effect, these policies become a kinder, clearer way of saying no. The beauty of personal policies is that they eliminate decision fatigue and offer clarity in moments of doubt. And they don't need to be perfect. As for so many others, for me, finding balance remains a perpetual tug-of-war. My instinct is to give equal attention to *everything* that matters to me. But to remind myself that I have limits, that I am important, I make a point of returning to my list of policies as a guide. My policies remind me of who I am, who I want to be, and the values that matter most to me. They help me prioritize myself and others and remind me that, as the saying goes, saying "no" to others is saying "yes" to ourselves.

Lead the revolution

Energized by her renewed sense of importance, Danna turned her attention to the countless teachers across the country struggling with the same exhaustion she had felt. She launched a monthly teacher support group she named "Happy Teacher Revolution." It's modeled after her lunches with Amanda and Heather and designed to make educators feel like a priority. The group is grounded in three principles: Self-care is essential, struggles and victories are to be shared, and boundaries are acts of strength. Their meetings, a mix of camaraderie and actionable advice, always end with optimism. Teachers share small wins or moments of joy, whether it's a student's breakthrough or the decision to leave work on time for once.

The group began modestly, with only a handful of teachers meeting in classrooms after hours. Then, as news of it spread, they started meeting in a church basement. Soon educators from neighboring schools—and even other districts—joined. Social media amplified the group's reach, with posts about teacher mental health resonating far beyond Danna's community. But the group's greatest impact was ensuring everyone who attended felt important and worthy of being prioritized. "This is a space where we can be ourselves," Danna said. "It's about making choices for our well-being and realizing we matter, not just as teachers but as people."

Today, Danna leads in-person and virtual workshops for teachers around the world, sharing the tools they need to establish their support systems at school. As one fifth-grade teacher put it, "They say you either survive or thrive when you become a teacher, but that was neither for me. I felt like I was dying." She went home crying every night, she continued, until in her third year, she discovered a community of support at Happy Teacher Revolution. "My job still causes stress, it is still chaotic, and I have

[bad] days," she said. "But I know how to handle them, how to embrace it, what to do to help me. And I have a group that will not let me do it alone."

At the end of *Mary Poppins*, Mary opens her umbrella and flies away, her work complete. Danna's impact is much the same. Wherever she goes, she leaves behind teachers who feel important, supported, and ready to nurture not only their students but also themselves and one another. I first came to Danna with questions about burnout, why it happens, and why it feels so unrelenting, but I left with something much deeper—a new appreciation for the transformative power of being prioritized. Importance, I learned, isn't just about being told you matter. It's about how others *show* you that you do.

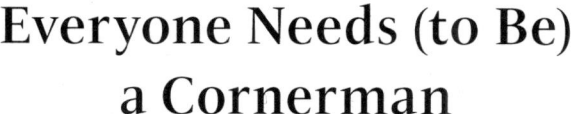

CHAPTER 4

Everyone Needs (to Be) a Cornerman

The Mattering Core

Recognition: You and your actions are valued, and your absence would be felt.

Reliance: You feel needed because others depend on you.

Importance: You feel significant because you're prioritized.

Ego Extension: You feel cared for because others are invested in your well-being.

Attunement: You feel deeply understood and meaningfully responded to.

Rehan Staton never could get used to the smell. Every bin he hauled into the tailgate of the garbage truck had a unique stench—of soiled diapers, spoiled milk, or the leftovers from a three-day-old steak dinner. In Bladensburg, Maryland, the sweltering days of August were the worst, worse than even the snow-storms of winter, Rehan told me over lunch, as other diners scooted around us with trays of salads and iced teas. Rehan spoke in a quiet, even tone, and occasionally, he'd look up as he recalled details from memories that stayed with him.

For hours, Rehan said, he would cling to the back of the garbage truck, catching the breeze when he could. They went house to house, stopping every couple dozen feet to throw the overflowing bags into the hopper. There was a decision to make in heat like this: to wear the protective gear and sweat half to death or stay slightly cooler and risk cutting your exposed arms on broken glass spilling out of a bag. On especially hot days, he said, most of the men opted for the latter, despite the fact that without protective gear, the stench would cling to their skin like a suffocating blanket.

Rehan never expected to be a sanitation worker. He grew up in a three-bedroom house with a backyard and a garage. His dad was a government IT contractor, and his mother was an assistant to a dental surgeon. Every discomfort had a remedy, he said. There was food for hunger, heat on cold days, and new shoes to replace worn-out ones. His father, with whom Rehan was closest, spent his spare time with Rehan and his brother, teaching them sports like tennis and martial arts.

Then, soon after his eighth birthday, life as he knew it changed. Rehan's mother abruptly left their family and returned to her native Sri Lanka. There had been signs she was unhappy, but her sudden departure caught her husband and sons by surprise. Soon after, Rehan's dad lost his job. To make ends meet, he took back-to-back shifts as a delivery driver. Food became scarce. Turning on the heat was now a luxury they couldn't afford, so they used the oven to warm the house. "I would have to sleep with a heavy jacket on when it was winter," said Rehan. He remembers waking up to the sight of his breath cutting through the cold.

Exhausted, hungry, and missing the active presence of his parents, Rehan fell behind in school. He couldn't concentrate and often feel asleep in class. He went from earning straight A's to placing near the bottom of his grade. Seeing his son struggle, Rehan's dad worked to get Rehan the academic help he needed. When Rehan started seventh grade, his dad went to a local community center to find a tutor. An aerospace engineer named Jamil offered to tutor Rehan free of charge. Rehan met him one-on-one a few times a week at the community center. Jamil found Rehan to be incredibly bright. With the right building blocks, Jamil told him, he could work in any field. Noticing Rehan's lack of basic necessities, Jamil bought him food and new shoes. They formulated game plans for tackling his schoolwork, and soon, Rehan made the honor roll.

But after several months, Jamil got a new assignment at work and had to end the tutoring. He gave Rehan a month's warning and promised to stay in touch. Rehan's father couldn't find another tutor willing to work for free, and there weren't enough hours left after his long workdays to help Rehan himself. So again, Rehan's grades suffered. His teachers began dismissing him as a disinterested student. One of them suggested he move to a special education track. Whatever motivation Rehan had dried up.

During his high school years, Rehan found his footing outside of the classroom. At a martial arts studio, he showed promise as a boxer, spending hours at a studio that let him train for free. After a few years, the trainer said he was talented enough to try to go pro. But Rehan faced another devastating setback his senior year when he developed tendonitis in both arms. Without insurance or access to physical therapy, Rehan was forced out of the ring. After bombing the SAT and being rejected by every college he applied to, Rehan had no clear path forward.

It was then that Rehan took a job at a local sanitation company. He worked alongside men who had been incarcerated, and others who, like him, lacked a college degree and had few opportunities. Rehan took pride in keeping his community clean, but it bothered him that people in the community ignored him, treating him as if he were unworthy of even basic recognition or respect. Worse than the feeling of invisibility was the sense of disdain he was sometimes forced to endure from strangers. Rehan recalled a time he was refurbishing old dumpsters one afternoon in a container yard in southeast Washington, DC. He overheard fragments of a conversation between a mother and her son who were walking past. The boy was curious about the roller brush Rehan was using to apply a fresh coat of paint. Then the mother's sharp voice cut through the humid air. "Don't end up like those men," she said, pointing to Rehan and a coworker.

As Rehan told me this story, he paused and set down his drink. Staring at the table, he said, "You never forget something like that."

Bet on people

Most of us will not face the humiliation Rehan experienced, but we can all relate to the painful feeling of being dismissed. You probably remember certain moments when your abilities were underestimated or ignored, like Ava, a New York mother who took a career pause to raise her children and found herself at a dinner party trying to share her thoughts on a political issue only to be met with a dismissive smile and a quick change of subject. Or Lisa, an executive assistant in California, who asked to learn more about her boss's work and felt rejected when he handed her a book about management from his bookshelf instead of discussing the work with her himself. Or Ken, who in retirement went to volunteer at a used bookstore that raised money for his Long Island, New York, town, but instead of being given real responsibilities, like choosing which books to put out and how to price them, he was assigned to be a door greeter. Ken told me that one of the hardest parts of getting older is that "people stop investing in you."

As painful as this kind of dismissal can be, it also suggests a more hopeful truth: that when we *do* have people in our lives who are invested in our growth, we're more likely to feel like we matter. You can probably remember someone whose interest in your unique capabilities changed the trajectory of your life, like that teacher who encouraged you to keep writing and gave you thoughtful feedback on draft after draft. Or an older brother who bought you a suit for your first job interview, saying, "I believe in you."

> *When you feel like you matter, you are secure in the knowledge that you have strong, meaningful connections to others and that you are not going through this life alone.*
>
> —Gordon Flett

Researchers call this aspect of mattering "ego extension," or the feeling that our successes and failures matter to someone else. It's one of the most powerful ways we understand our connection to others. As researcher Morris Rosenberg noted, ego extension works both ways. For both the giver and the recipient, ego extension is about feeling part of something larger than yourself, knowing that you have an important role to play in someone else's life and that they play an important role in yours. The joys, struggles, and experiences of another person broaden your inner world. Their happiness becomes your happiness; their heartache, your heartache. The knowledge that we are part of others' lives makes us feel valued. With ego extension, we both grow—and extend—beyond ourselves.

Ego extension also creates a bond of accountability. When someone is invested in us, we want to make them proud. We care about disappointing them. Early in life, the people we typically feel that investment from are our parents and teachers. Studies conducted by the National Center for Education Statistics readily show this dynamic: When students have adults in their lives who believe and invest in them, they tend to have higher grades, show increased motivation, and experience greater success. One study among 140 "at-risk" ninth graders in the Midwest found that students were less inclined to drop out of school when they had relationships with adult tutors who cared not only about their success in academics but also about their success in life.

By contrast, when we lack people in our lives who express a vested interest in us, we can lose our sense of possibility. We may have our own personal vision boards and goals, but without people on the sidelines cheering us on, encouraging us through setbacks, and holding us accountable, we might start to doubt our capabilities. We lose confidence when we hit road bumps, grow stagnant, or play small.

When I first met Rehan, I was immediately struck by his determination. While humble, he carried himself in a way that made it clear he was going places. It was obvious he had so much potential, so much to offer the world. But potential alone isn't enough. Without a strong network of people invested in our success—people who see our future as worth nurturing—it's easy to lack confidence or give up.

Rehan knew his father cared deeply about his future. But he needed this ego extension from other people, too, like Jamil, his tutor, or his martial arts coach. He didn't blame the teachers in his large public high school for their inability to provide him with this investment. "They had to support so many young people that it must have been overwhelming to help me through my family's struggles and my academic challenges," he said.

Still, it stung when life told him that he had no potential, like when people handled their waste so carelessly, throwing their broken glass, needles, and knives into trash bags with no regard for the person who was going to pick them up. Over time, Rehan began to internalize this disregard, like the way people avoided eye contact when he was in his work uniform and how they held their breath as they hurried past, as if his very presence carried with it the stench of the work he did.

Invite them into the ring

One of Rehan's main jobs at the sanitation company was refurbishing old dumpsters, including picking off anything that had stuck to the smelly containers. "You never knew what you were going to find," he said. In one dumpster, a coworker once found a grenade. Another found a human hand stuck to the bottom. The refurbishing process was notoriously grueling. Each dumpster was addressed piecemeal. Workers would remove stickers or debris from one side, then clean or sand that same section before moving on to the next.

Rehan saw the inefficiency of this process and decided to try a new approach. First, rip everything off all sides of the dumpster—stickers, labels, and debris—in one go. Then, sand down the entire surface thoroughly, ensuring a clean and uniform base. Finally, paint the dumpster in one smooth, uninterrupted step. By batching tasks together, Rehan eliminated the constant tool switching and backtracking that had bogged down the old system. The first day he tried out the method, Rehan and a coworker knocked out seven cans in a day. The usual tally was two, at most four. "Seven was unheard of," he told me.

Two of Rehan's coworkers, Bones and Craig, quickly took a liking to Rehan for his work ethic and ingenuity. Both men were a decade older and were a bit of an odd couple: Bones was short and skinny, while Craig was extremely tall and big. Bones never talked about his past. Craig had served time in prison for a drug-related crime. He had once been shot in the face, but thanks to a skilled surgeon, no one could tell except when he took his fake teeth out before he ate. The two men treated Rehan like a son. Every day, they built Rehan up with compliments by telling him, "You're smart, thoughtful, a hard worker, and a really good kid." They told him that he had things to offer the world. "You need to go to college," they often told him.

With Bones's and Craig's constant validation, Rehan started walking a little taller. Still, his grades were terrible, and his test scores were worse. What college would ever take him? But Bones and Craig would hear none of this. One day they marched into the front office to speak with the company owner's son, Brent. "Let's find this guy something to do that is not here," they pleaded. Rehan needed to go to college. "He's too smart for this." Brent, who had known Rehan's family for years, agreed. The following week, he drove Rehan to meet with a counselor at nearby Bowie State University. The counselor asked Rehan a lot of questions. It was true that, on paper, Rehan appeared to have little promise, but the counselor liked how inquisitive and obviously hardworking he was. He told Rehan to submit an appeal to the admissions committee.

Within a few weeks, he was admitted. The counselor gave Rehan access to free tutors and a partial scholarship to cover his tuition. Rehan's family and colleagues rallied around him. The first semester, his dad worked overtime to help cover tuition so Rehan could take fewer shifts at work and get his bearings as a student. For the second semester, the sanitation department scheduled his shifts around his class schedule. Rehan woke up at four a.m., worked until nine a.m., headed to school, and then worked a late-afternoon shift. It wasn't easy. Occasionally he slid into class late, sitting in the back of the classroom to avoid judgmental glances when he hadn't had time to shower after his morning shift. When the heat wasn't on at home, he headed back to campus at night, searching for warm places to study.

Rehan finished his first semester with a 3.7 GPA, but by the end of the second semester, his grades were dropping precipitously. It was so hard to juggle work and school. But Rehan didn't want to let his dad down, or Brent or Bones and Craig. He knew how proud they were. Brent stayed close, buying Rehan food and checking in to make sure his work schedule didn't overwhelm him. Rehan found the courage to ask his teachers for help, something he'd never done before. Could deadlines for papers be extended? Were there study strategies they recommended? To his surprise, his teachers responded enthusiastically and offered specific advice. They showed him how to use class notes to predict test questions so he could focus on the material most likely to appear on exams. One teacher suggested Rehan send him outlines and early drafts of his essays for feedback. Armed with these strategies, Rehan restructured his approach to school. The results were striking. By sophomore year, he had finished both semesters with a perfect 4.0 GPA.

The counselor who'd admitted Rehan urged him to take on a bigger challenge, to apply to transfer to the University of Maryland. Rehan was accepted for his junior year. But then came a major blow. His dad suffered a stroke, which made him unable to work. Rehan would need to earn extra money now to care for his father. He wasn't sure he could sustain his academics. Once again, others stepped in to help. In one particularly difficult moment, a professor gave Rehan two hundred dollars to get him through the week. Other professors extended office hours so Rehan could meet around his work schedule. Brent consistently checked in. Rehan felt a new resolve. He couldn't bear to disappoint anyone after so many kindnesses had been offered to him. "If this were just about me and just fighting for myself, I definitely would have quit," he said.

The simple power of having someone "in your corner," listening to you, taking an interest in you, entering into your life from the outside and caring, does wonders for a suffering person.

—John Z.

Rehan thrived academically and as a class leader. He served as president of the undergraduate history association, and by senior year, he had been invited to the Dean's Advisory Board with the university's trustees as the only student on the committee. When people asked what he wanted to do after college, he told them he was planning to attend Harvard Law School. Rehan said this wasn't an achievable goal, really, not with his work demands or the need to support his dad. But he liked the symbol of what he could be, of what he could reach for. He thought of how Bones and Craig helped unlock a future when so many others hadn't seen anything in him. "It was the sanitation workers who saw me and lifted me up," he said.

The fall of his senior year, Rehan auditioned to be the winter commencement speaker and, to his surprise, was selected. That

December, Rehan spoke to more than 4,700 classmates, using his experience in boxing as a metaphor for life goals. "No fighter steps into the ring alone," Rehan said. "Every boxer has a cornerman." The cornerman is much more than just a coach who stands beyond the ropes, he explained. It is the person who knows the boxer's strengths, vulnerabilities, and capacities better than anyone else. The cornerman sees the fight from an outside perspective, allowing them to give the fighter honest advice, and is deeply, personally invested in the fighter's success. Most importantly, a cornerman offers the reminder that you're not in the fight alone. "A good cornerman," Rehan said, "is the difference between giving up and finding that extra push to keep going."

The same is true outside the ring, Rehan continued. The reason he was standing there that day was because of the many cornermen in his life. The professors who regularly checked in on him. The counselor who made sure he was on track. The coworkers who made sure his trash shifts worked with his class schedule. His dad, who cared so deeply whether he succeeded. We all need cornermen in our lives, said Rehan, and we need to be cornermen for others, because life can deal us all sorts of defeats. "A champion is someone who gets back up," he said. "We are champions because we pick each other up."

Accept investment

Over the years, I've been lucky to have many trusted cornermen in my life. As a new parent, I left my job at *60 Minutes* to be the primary caregiver. Years later, with my three children in elementary school, I went back to work. With the travel demands of television production, going back to *60 Minutes* wouldn't work for our family. But maybe, I thought, I could carve out something for myself in print journalism. Then self-doubt seeped in. *What print editor wants to hire an out-of-work TV journalist? I haven't written a newspaper article since my college days. Would I even know what to do?* The negative thoughts were paralyzing.

Over dinner, I opened up to Katie and Tira, two close friends I'd met years earlier while at *60 Minutes.* Katie, who was a working parent, encouraged me to put myself back in the ring: "You're a seasoned journalist, and you don't lose that by taking a few years off." Katie then challenged me further. "If you're serious, we're going to hold you accountable," she said. "Next month, come to our dinner with three story pitches." In our weekly phone calls, she checked in to see how my "assignment" was going, emailed me potential story ideas, and stayed firm with her "deadline." When I presented the pitches at our next dinner, she and Tira offered me useful feedback: "What about this angle? What about interviewing this person?" They helped me brainstorm where to send the pitches and proofread my emails to editors. When my first article was accepted by *The Wall Street Journal*, Katie and Tira took me to dinner to celebrate.

As the sanitation workers did for Rehan and as Katie and Tira did for me, trusted cornermen see and name what we are capable of when we can't see it ourselves. In boxing, no one did it better than Angelo Dundee, arguably the greatest cornerman of all time. Over his fifty-year career, he worked with many of the world's most legendary boxers, including Muhammad Ali and Sugar Ray

Leonard. Dundee's talent wasn't his boxing technique. It was the connection he built with his fighters. That connection was never more critical than during Leonard's legendary 1981 fight, dubbed "The Showdown," against Tommy Hearns for the undisputed welterweight championship. Hearns won the early rounds. Leonard rallied in the middle rounds to briefly regain momentum until Hearns took back control. When Leonard returned to his corner after the twelfth round, fatigued and with his left eye nearly swollen shut, Dundee put a steadying hand on his shoulder and said urgently, "You're blowing it, son. You're blowing it!"

Dundee's words weren't criticism. They were the words of someone who believed Leonard still had it in him to win. "When he said it," Leonard later recalled, "I knew what I had to do." In the thirteenth round, Leonard unleashed a series of punches that left Hearns dazed. Ultimately, the referee was forced to stop the fight. Leonard's comeback remains one of boxing's greatest victories— and it wouldn't have happened without Dundee's unwavering belief in him.

What Dundee did for Leonard is what all good cornermen do for their fighters. They remind us of our potential, even when we can't see it for ourselves. Our "cornermen" protect our sense of mattering by affirming who we are now and who we can be in the future. Like Dundee, they allow us to borrow their courage when we feel like we're on the ropes. Cornermen are uniquely positioned to see what we might not be able to see, the hidden talents and vulnerabilities that we might not fully see in ourselves. And they are brave enough to call them out, even when it's uncomfortable.

Unlike a cheerleader who only offers encouragement, a cornerman is willing to tell us what we *need* to hear, just as Dundee saw that Leonard needed to hear that he was "blowing it."

The cornermen in my life know that my "love language" is honest feedback. To me, there's no greater gift or act of love and support than a friend willing to be open and vulnerable enough to tell me what I need to hear. To me, hard truths delivered with care are the ultimate sign of someone's investment in me. To invite this kind of help—to welcome someone into our corner—requires openness and humility. We have to be willing to listen and take in the feedback they offer. After all, their support can only go as far as we let it. When we're open to their guidance, cornermen do more than urge us on—they help us grow into who we're meant to be.

Where to look

We don't have to wait for cornermen to appear in our lives. We can actively search for them. There are the obvious places, like among our more senior coworkers or family members. But potential cornermen are all around us. Maybe it's a neighbor who always asks thoughtful questions, a former teacher who saw something in us long before we did, or a friend who always celebrates others' wins. Finding the right people often begins with noticing how you feel in their presence: Do they make you feel more like yourself, or do their words leave you less secure? Healthy encouragement helps us grow without making us feel inadequate in the process.

Many of us hesitate to welcome this kind of investment. Maybe we've internalized the false ideal of self-reliance. Perhaps we worry that we are unworthy of their help or are concerned that an ask is a burden. Or maybe we believe that most relationships are transactional and that people only help those who can help them back. Maybe we are worried that asking for insight and investment might reveal that we don't actually have potential. In my first year at *60 Minutes*, I was juggling the high expectations of working at a prestigious show and the pressure of proving myself in a new role. I was determined to establish my competence and earn my place. So when the learning curve felt steep, I kept my head down and pushed through, brushing aside offers of help from colleagues. Accepting help, I feared, would somehow expose me as unqualified or incapable.

Once I was assigned to research and fact-check a particularly complex story. The deadline was tight, and I was struggling to get it done. Phil, a legendary senior producer, casually stopped by my windowless closet of an office to offer his support, saying, "If you need a fresh set of eyes, I'm here." I remember feeling a twinge of relief at the thought of sharing the load, but my inner critic won out. *If you ask for help, you'll look incompetent.* So I smiled and declined. "Thanks, Phil, but I think I've got this." I was determined to figure it out alone. Looking back, not only did I lose out on practical support, I also lost out on Phil's subtle offer to invest in me. I was so narrowly focused on proving my competence that I couldn't see that bigger picture.

The truth is, we often misplace our fears about seeking help.

"Miscalibrated expectation" is what researchers have termed the phenomenon of how much we underestimate the willingness of others to help us and how good the help-giver will feel afterward. When we need help, we tend to overestimate human selfishness and underestimate the innate generosity that is wired within us. But we can recalibrate by taking steps to invite others in. It can start by asking for feedback on a project or reaching out for a small piece of advice. Each act reminds us that we are worthy of support. Over time, I learned to push through my fear of accepting help. One day, Phil passed by my office and asked what I was working on. I told him about a story I was researching and asked for his take. He listened, then offered to connect me with someone who could offer deeper insight. This interaction showed me that inviting someone in doesn't diminish us. It actually does the opposite. Letting others in is how we become stronger and wiser.

Rehan knew that he made it through college thanks to the investment of his many cornermen. After graduation, however, Rehan received another blow when his health suddenly began to deteriorate. Severe fatigue, persistent shortness of breath, and sharp chest pains left him struggling to get through the day. Rehan didn't seek medical attention because he couldn't afford it. Instead, he rested in bed, hoping the mysterious illness would pass.

In Rehan's moment of crisis, his cornermen helped him see a path through. Rehan's cousin Dominic visited regularly, bringing him food, water, and medicine. On the days when Dominic wasn't working his shift at Dunkin' Donuts, he sat beside Rehan for hours while he studied for the LSAT. When the symptoms flared, Dominic helped mitigate them, rubbing his back and encouraging him to drink water, so Rehan could go back to studying. One day, Rehan ran out of money and could no longer afford food. Unbeknownst to Rehan, Dominic spent his last seven dollars buying Rehan a box of organic strawberries. "Why organic?" Rehan asked him in amazement and gratitude. Dominic said that he worried the pesticides could cause Rehan to have a reaction.

While Rehan never discovered the source of his sickness, he recovered with rest. From his bed, Rehan applied to the country's best law schools and, at twenty-four, was accepted into many of his top choices: USC, Columbia, and the University of Pennsylvania. Then, when Rehan opened the email to find out he'd gotten into Harvard Law School, Dominic was right there with him, cheering and smiling from ear to ear. The victory wasn't just Rehan's success; it was *their* success.

Be a cornerman

There are moments in life that break you open. For me, one of those came on July 25, 2023, when my beloved cornerman, Katie, passed away after a five-year battle with ovarian cancer. I had the honor of eulogizing Katie at a standing-room-only mass at her church in New Jersey. At the lectern, I asked everyone to raise their hand if they considered Katie one of their most trusted friends, someone who was deeply invested in them. Nearly every hand in the church went up. "How can one person touch so many lives?" I asked, amazed. Katie brought out the best in everyone around her and reveled in her friends' joys like they were her own. On a sad or hard day, there was no greater guide, strategizing ways to help and reminding you that you'll get through it. When Katie was your cornerman, you wanted to be worthy of her investment.

Before her death, Katie, two other friends, and I brought together a small group to form a women-in-media dinner circle. We wanted to create a space where women could gather for mutual investment, a place where we could ask for professional help and offer help to others. We launched it right before Katie died, but she was too sick to attend the first event. After her death, deep in grief, I decided there was no better way to honor Katie's legacy as cornerman extraordinaire than to continue with these dinners. So that's exactly what we did. Every few months, a handful of women gather to share a meal. We talk about personal and professional struggles, our goals, our setbacks, and our fears. The real magic of the dinner comes at the end of the evening. In the last twenty minutes of our conversation, we go around the table and open up about something we could use help with. The group offers feedback and guidance. By formalizing asking for help, we normalize it. Actually, we insist on it. You're not allowed to pass. Katie would have loved it. These dinners have become a way to carry on Katie's legacy as a cornerman, supporting one another just as she supported so many.

Offer your time, talent, and treasure

To be a cornerman, we don't need to wipe our calendars clean or hold special credentials. What matters most is our willingness to be there for others with whatever we have to give. A simple place to begin is by asking, Who in your life could use your three T's—time, talent, and treasure? Maybe it's someone in your book club who recently lost a loved one and would appreciate a weekly walk. That's time. Treasure includes any resources you might have, perhaps offering your car for a friend's doctor's appointment or lending unused office space to someone starting a business. Talent means sharing your unique skills to support someone else's goal, like using your marketing know-how to help a friend launch their nonprofit or mentoring a student in your field. Being a cornerman is about doing what you can, with what you have, to support someone.

This is precisely what Emily did. When Emily moved to Boston after college, her life seemed full of excitement: a new job as a data scientist, a big city, and fresh experiences. But beneath the surface, she felt deeply lonely, missing the friendships she'd left behind. One evening, she stumbled on a video of a visually impaired runner crossing a Paralympic finish line with his guide from Achilles International, an organization that pairs guides with disabled athletes. Emily had always loved running and, inspired by the organization's work, she signed up as a volunteer. She was partnered with a young man named Justin. Diagnosed as a child with muscular dystrophy along with a serious spinal complication, Justin was told he would likely never walk independently, let alone run. But through years of determination, physical therapy, and sheer grit, Justin defied expectations by taking his first unassisted steps and eventually discovering a love for distance running. Now, he was training for the Boston Marathon.

Initially, their partnership was practical. Emily's job was to help Justin train for the course by pacing their runs and offering encouragement. Soon, however, Emily found herself thinking about Justin's progress outside their training sessions. She started checking her weather app more often, ensuring favorable conditions for their next practice run. She developed a training plan to accommodate Justin's work schedule as a greeter at a hotel. Emily researched techniques to help him balance and held him accountable by ensuring he was following the plan and taking necessary rest days. Even after long days at her job, she fine-tuned their training schedule to help him edge closer to his race-day goal.

With time, Justin's successes and struggles on their practice runs began to feel like her own. "We need to work on that hill," she'd say, or, "We're getting stronger." When Justin struggled on Boston's famous "Heartbreak Hill," Emily felt his frustration in her muscles, too. When he hit a personal record, she beamed with pride. One chilly afternoon, after a particularly grueling run, Justin turned to Emily, sweat soaking through his shirt, and said, "I know sometimes I seem mad at you when you are challenging me to do better, but I am so thankful for you, bestie. You are like a sister to me, and I couldn't have done this without you." At that moment, Emily realized that their connection was mutual; Justin welcomed her dedication.

After months of training, race day arrived. The weather was cool and overcast, and bursts of torrential rain made the streets slippery. Justin began to struggle halfway through the race, suffering serious pain and muscle tightness. But he wanted to push through, so he told her, "I'm hurting really bad, but we got this, bestie. Let's show them what I am made of." Without hesitation, Emily reached for his hand. For the next thirteen miles, the two ran together, hand in hand. Running this way required Emily to adjust her stride constantly, counterbalancing Justin's movements while maintaining her own footing. Her hand and arm cramped, her shoulder ached, and her knee throbbed, all while the rain soaked through their clothes. But she brushed off the pain. Their goal overpowered everything else. When they crossed the finish line, Justin had set a new personal record: 05:31:38. Emily threw her arms around him. The rain mixed with the tears of joy rolling down her cheek. Justin's triumph felt like hers, too.

Share their joy

One of the best ways to show our investment in someone is to celebrate their successes as if they were our own. Many people, especially those who are high-achieving, tend to breeze past their milestones, already focusing on their next goal, without really pausing to see how far they've come. That's where a trusted cornerman comes in. Taking time to savor another person's success with them—to see it, name it, and make a point to celebrate it— offers recognition, importance, and ego extension all rolled up into one gesture.

> To get the full value of joy, you must have someone to divide it with.
>
> —Mark Twain

When we relish someone else's joy, something meaningful happens to us, too. Neuroimaging studies find that witnessing others' positive experiences actually activates our own reward-related regions of the brain. In other words, their success becomes our success; their joy, our joy. There's a name for this kind of shared experience. In Buddhist tradition, it's called *mudita,* or the pleasure we take in another's well-being. It is the belief that joy and achievement are abundant and that there's plenty to go around. This concept offers a radical alternative in a competitive culture that often teaches us to view success as zero-sum, where another's achievement can feel like a subtraction from our own. When someone receives good news, a person practicing mudita feels authentic delight rather than comparison or resentment.

Mudita doesn't deny envy's existence. Instead, it provides a more generous and constructive way to respond to it. Envy is a universal human response with evolutionary roots. For our early ancestors, it served a purpose, directing our attention to what others had that might be essential for survival. We don't have to judge ourselves for feeling envy, but we do have to hold ourselves accountable for how we respond to it. When feelings of envy bubble up, research shows we face a choice. We can follow the route of what psychologists call "malicious envy," which tempts us to undercut others to feel better by comparison. Or we can take the "benign envy" route, which allows another's success to inspire us instead.

But what if we could go even further than inspiration? What if we could transform that initial pang of "I wish I had what they have" into "How can I help them succeed even more?" This is where mudita connects to ego extension. When we practice mudita—taking genuine joy in others' success—we're already beginning to stretch our sense of self beyond our individual boundaries. Ego extension invites us to take this one step further, to become an active participant in someone else's growth and success. When we make this kind of investment, their growth becomes part of our identity, too, stretching our sense of self to include the lives we've helped shape. As we help others grow into who they are meant to be, we become more of who we are meant to be, too.

Accompany them in hardship

Physician Paul Farmer was renowned for transforming healthcare systems in some of the world's most struggling communities. He cofounded Partners In Health, an organization that brought high-quality care to places where many believed it impossible, such as rural Haiti, war-torn Rwanda, and Siberian prisons. Rather than accepting limited resources as an excuse for inadequate care, Farmer built systems that treated patients with the same dignity as those in the world's wealthiest hospitals. In his work, Farmer embraced the philosophy of "accompaniment," a deeply relational approach rooted in the Spanish *compañero*, meaning "friend," and the Latin *ad cum panis*, "to break bread together." Farmer believed that true support meant accompanying people, walking beside them, offering solidarity, and sharing their burdens and fate for a while. This kind of presence is a powerful form of ego extension. When we accompany others, like a cornerman in a fight, we are able to offer them steady, ongoing support through their struggles. Our presence says to them they're not alone and they don't have to be at their best to be worthy of care. It also reminds us that we don't have to fix something to make a meaningful difference in the world around us.

Accompaniment asks something intimate and difficult, that we sit with someone's pain rather than dismiss or try to repair it. When faced with a loved one's challenges, it's natural to want to minimize their feelings ("It's okay, don't worry") or jump into problem-solving mode ("What if you tried . . . ?"). But accompaniment requires a pause, a willingness to feel their hurt alongside them. And just as important, it asks us not to move on too quickly. In everyday life, accompaniment shows up in small gestures, like making a meal for a tired friend or sending a text just to say "I'm checking in on you," a signal that they aren't alone.

It can include offering what you might think of as "invisible" and "surprise" support. Invisible support is the hidden efforts to alleviate someone's burdens, such as managing household chores, entertaining the kids, or preparing a favorite comfort meal during a difficult time for a partner. Surprise support offers encouragement in unexpected ways, like sending flowers before an interview or leaving an encouraging note on someone's desk. Opportunities to provide this type of care can be found in friendships, families, workplaces, and communities. The challenge is to notice them and have the courage to push through any discomfort to offer that support. As Farmer has said, "Everyone who draws breath needs accompaniment."

The Reciprocity Effect

Rehan started Harvard Law School during the pandemic in the fall of 2020. The following year, when Rehan finally moved onto campus, the transition was strange, he said. His classmates were warm and welcoming, but Rehan felt acutely aware of the difference in their backgrounds. Classmates talked about heading to Europe just for the weekend, while Rehan didn't even have a passport.

One day while walking down a hall on campus, Rehan passed a custodian and asked how she was doing. She stared at him blankly. He politely asked again. "I'm sorry—I didn't know you were talking to me," she told him. "Students would usually rather look at the wall than talk to me." Rehan flashed back to his time on the garbage truck, when he was written off by everyone except the men in the truck alongside him. He recognized his own past mattering struggle in the custodian.

As he went about the rest of his day, that conversation with the custodian stayed with him. Rehan was curious. Did all support staff at Harvard feel this sense of disconnection from the rest of the community on campus? He began seeking out campus custodians, security guards, and dining hall attendants to see if they shared the woman's view. He asked them, "Do you feel supported by the school? Do you feel appreciated by the students?" Brione, who has worked in catering for Harvard Law School for twenty-two years, recalled at first being mistrustful of Rehan and all his questions. "What's this guy's angle? What is he trying to get by asking me all these questions?" Then he heard Rehan's backstory and realized, "Oh, he's one of us. Now I get it."

Rehan found that staff members he spoke with described feeling unseen, too. "When students brush past us," one support staff member told him, "no one says excuse me." Brione echoed this sentiment when I met him on campus, noting, "No one notices the windows when they are clean or the pathways when they are cleared after an overnight snowstorm. Most students don't realize that there's a person working hard to clean that glass to keep their environment clean."

Rehan decided he wanted to change this attitude and show his appreciation to the workers by using his savings from a summer job at a law firm to buy Amazon gift cards for one hundred support staff members at Harvard Law School, which he personally delivered inside handwritten thank-you cards. The response from the staff was overwhelming. Many of them emphasized how wonderful it felt to finally be "seen" by a student. "Not only does he notice," Brione told me about Rehan, "he appreciates us and reciprocates with kindness."

But Rehan didn't stop there. Along with a few other students, he spent months planning a party in honor of the support staff that would bring the Harvard community together in gratitude. Two hundred people attended, including support staff and their families, students, and a few faculty members. The students served dinner while the support staff celebrated. Bates Trucking & Trash Removal, Rehan's former employer, donated money to cover expenses and provide gift cards for the staff. As part of the celebration, the team handed out various awards, voted on by both students and the support staff themselves, recognizing contributions that often went unseen.

After the party, Rehan and other student volunteers continued to show their appreciation. They regularly engaged in letter-writing campaigns in which students sent notes of appreciation to the staff. Brione said that after the awards ceremony and appreciation campaigns, staff members walked with their heads held higher, feeling for the first time that they were not only important members of the community but also genuinely invested in. When Rehan graduated, other students stepped up to expand on his efforts, including involving the Harvard Law School Student Government to keep what had become known as "the Reciprocity Effect" alive. Rehan has remained involved even after graduation, helping secure nonprofit status and partnering with other clubs to keep these ceremonies going.

Rehan recognized something in the support staff at Harvard. It was the same feeling he once had while working for the sanitation company. They felt written off, unseen by the very community they served. And just as he had longed for acknowledgment in his own work, he took it upon himself to help restore their sense of mattering. In doing so, something shifted for Rehan, too. By lifting others up, he reinforced his own sense of purpose. He didn't just pass through Harvard. He left a mark.

Today, Rehan lives in New York and works at one of the country's most prestigious law firms. Soon after he started his job, his father unexpectedly passed away from a heart attack. The loss was staggering. Months later, when we met in person, the grief was seared into his face. But Rehan's face softened when he recalled how his strong network of friends and mentors helped see him through the tragedy. At the funeral, the cornermen who helped him through the most difficult periods of his life returned to yet again offer their support. His seventh-grade tutor, who had been the first to recognize his potential, made the journey. Bones and Brent, who were a steady presence in his life, were there, too. His counselor at Bowie State, who guided Rehan through those pivotal college years, attended. These people had stayed in his life over years, or in some cases decades. Their investment stretched beyond any one chapter of his life.

Rehan finds it hard to imagine a life without his father, but he's relying, as ever, on his cornermen. He's confident in his ability to persevere, he said, "not because I'm great but because my team is great." He added, "I have never viewed myself as a pick-myself-up-by-the-bootstraps kind of guy, and I see no honor in being a self-made man." Just then, the competitive spark of the old boxer in him came alive: "What I know is that if I have to compete against a self-made man, it should be easy to win because of the incredible team I have with me in the ring."

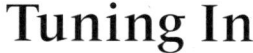

CHAPTER 5

Tuning In

> ## The Mattering Core
>
> **Recognition:** You and your actions are valued, and your absence would be felt.
>
> **Reliance:** You feel needed because others depend on you.
>
> **Importance:** You feel significant because you're prioritized.
>
> **Ego Extension:** You feel cared for because others are invested in your well-being.
>
> **Attunement: You feel deeply understood and meaningfully responded to.**

At four thirty a.m., an Uber driver navigated me through a quiet neighborhood in St. Louis. All of the houses were dark, except for one. As we pulled up to it, two large dogs barked behind the door. Seconds later it swung open, and Peggy Winckowski greeted me with a big, warm smile, all while holding back the excited dogs that weighed more than she did.

Peggy quietly led me down the hallway toward the kitchen. As we passed the downstairs master bedroom, she reached out to gently close the door because her husband, who has Parkinson's and dementia, was still asleep. Peggy had already started on breakfast. On the counter were five egg cartons, five pounds of uncooked bacon, two jumbo-sized loaves of bread, and fresh fruit. "Teenage boys eat like they've been starved for weeks," Peggy joked. It was an extraordinary sight to see so much food, but perhaps what was most extraordinary was how casual Peggy was about it all, as if waking up at four a.m. to cook pounds of bacon was no big deal.

The tradition started in October 2021, when her grandson Sam, then a freshman at Bishop DuBourg High School, and his friends met for breakfast at a local diner before their late-start Wednesdays. Sam told them, "My Grandma Peggy makes a better breakfast than this." Then he added, "You guys should really come over to her house instead." That casual invitation turned into a weekly tradition, now known as the Wednesday Breakfast Club.

On the morning I was there, just before seven a steady stream of teens trickled in with backpacks slung across their shoulders. They beelined directly to the kitchen, where Grandma Peggy—as they all called her—greeted each of them with a warm, one-armed hug as she skillfully flipped bacon with the other. It was clear right away that Peggy knew them well—not just their names but what was going on in their lives, like who had a dreaded chemistry test that day, who was worried about making varsity, who was still healing from a painful breakup, and who was working hard to break his vaping habit. And they knew her, too. One girl asked how her garden was holding up after the recent storm, and another asked about Peggy's husband.

At one point mid-meal, Peggy paused and looked around the table, flushed with pride. "I just love you kids," she said, beaming. After breakfast, I asked a few of the teens what these mornings meant to them. One told me, "It just feels really good to be here." Another girl, in a soccer hoodie, took a moment before saying, "I think it's knowing someone is always happy to see you." Peggy nodded. "We feed each other," she said.

As I watched the teens and Peggy eat and talk, it became clear to me that what made these mornings special wasn't the food (although it was delicious). It was the way Peggy paid attention. She noticed things without anyone saying a word, like who seemed off that day, who was under a lot of stress, and who needed a little extra attention. Peggy was tuned in to the signals of these young people. That kind of emotional precision, her ability to notice and provide care without being asked, is rare. What made these mornings powerful was what psychologists call "attunement," or the practice of making people feel understood.

Tune in

Picture coming home after a long, exhausting day. You drop your keys on the counter, and when your partner asks how you're doing, you give an automatic response: "I'm fine." Rather than simply accepting your response and moving on, your partner notices the slight hesitation in your voice. They pause to examine your face and say, "What's wrong? Did that conversation with your boss not go the way you hoped?" In that moment, you let out the breath you didn't realize you were holding. The tension in your shoulders starts to ease. Your partner didn't just sense that something was off—they understood what it was. And suddenly, you don't feel so alone.

That is the feeling of attunement, the fifth component to building our mattering core. It assures us that someone "gets us." Attunement is like salt in a Thanksgiving dinner, a subtle but transformative ingredient. Without it, even the most thoughtful mattering strategies can feel bland or incomplete. Attunement allows you to respond to the nuances of a moment and ensures that your efforts to make someone feel valued actually land in a way that feels right to them. It is the difference between seeing someone and seeking to understand them.

For example, consider how you might support a grieving friend by drawing on the different threads of the mattering core. Recognition would mean seeing their pain and acknowledging their struggle. Reliance might move you to bring a meal or run errands. Importance could mean rearranging your schedule to be there for them. Ego extension might look like investing in their wellbeing by finding them a support group. But attunement goes deeper— it's about understanding what they need emotionally in this moment and offering support in a way that truly meets them where they are. "When we attune to others, we allow our own internal state to shift, to come to resonate with the inner world of another," writes psychiatrist Dan Siegel. "This resonance is at the heart of the important sense of 'feeling felt' that emerges in close relationships."

Mattering without a sense of attunement can feel hollow, like offering a gift that misses the mark because we didn't take the time to understand what the other person really liked or wanted. Instead of relying on a one-size-fits-all approach, it prompts us to pay specific attention. Does my friend need words or silence? Distraction or space? A hug, a home-cooked meal, or just someone to sit with them? Attunement provides the kind of comfort that truly resonates. The psychologist Richard Erskine called attunement "a kinesthetic and emotional sensing of others" by "metaphorically being in their skin." In other words, it is the capacity to be in sync with another person's inner world.

By contrast, a lack of attunement can feel isolating. It's something most of us have felt, like being half listened to or misunderstood. It's when someone asks, "How are you?" but is already looking down at their phone before you can answer. Or perhaps you're sharing something painful, and then the other person interrupts with their own story. While they may mean well, the interruption keeps the connection shallow, and the opportunity for attunement is lost. What's tricky is that in our busy daily lives these small moments are easy to overlook.

> *Attention is the rarest and purest form of generosity.*
>
> —Simone Weil

Our sense of self is shaped, in part, by the ways others reflect us back to ourselves, and without those mirrors, we can start to feel like radio signals with no receivers, broadcasting our thoughts, emotions, and needs into the void. When our signal is routinely missed, we might stop opening up to friends or loved ones because we feel like we will be ignored. What starts as self-preservation—choosing to retreat—can slowly strip away the joy of being seen, heard, and valued.

Psychologist Edward Tronick's famous "Still Face" experiment demonstrates the profound impact of this kind of misattunement. In this study, a mother first engages warmly with her baby, reflecting the baby's emotions through expressions and touch. Then, she abruptly stops responding. Her expression goes blank. It's a break in attunement. The baby, who depends on the mother's emotional feedback, initially tries to reengage by smiling, cooing, or reaching out. When the mother remains unresponsive, frustration sets in and the baby shows signs of distress. If the caregiver remains unresponsive, eventually the baby may shut down and detach emotionally. This experiment shows us why attunement matters. It reassures us that our emotions—and by extension that we—are worthy of a connected response. Over time, repeated experiences of misattunement can lead children to internalize shame, forming the belief that their emotions are too much, or worse, that maybe *they* are somehow unworthy of love and connection. The same dynamic can play out in adulthood. When our words, emotions, or needs go unnoticed or are dismissed, we can begin to turn inward and shut down ourselves.

If attention is our most valuable resource, then tuning in is one of the best ways to show someone they matter. Like any skill, attunement can either strengthen with practice or atrophy without use. Our modern lives are filled with so much input, endless notifications, social media, emails, and interruptions that we often struggle to find the bandwidth to attune to each other. I know this challenge personally. It's in moments when I catch myself half listening that I try to refocus. It takes intentional effort to slow down enough to notice someone else's signals. But it's that extra effort that feels so valuable to the person on the receiving end. Like any practice, the more we make a habit of truly *tuning in*, the more natural it becomes.

Fight inertia

To get proficient in attunement, we need to spend time together in person. It matters more than we might realize. Video calls and texting help us stay in touch. However, they don't give us access to the full range of human signals we rely on to feel understood and cared for, like noticing someone's subtle hesitation before they speak or that they're moving slower than usual. These cues—tone of voice, facial expressions, and body language—are how we read someone's inner landscape.

Modern life makes it so much easier to stay home and miss these opportunities. With a few taps, we can order dinner, stream anything we want, chat from the couch, and avoid the friction of putting on shoes, facing bad weather, or having to make draining small talk. Also, in the long shadow of the pandemic, staying home now feels normal.

Bailing, Flaking, Canceling: In a 2023 survey by the American Psychological Association, 25 percent of respondents admitted to canceling social plans in the last month. The next time you're inclined to cancel, consider how your mattering might be better supported if you said yes instead. How about the mattering of others? "Just a reminder that when you cancel plans with someone who lives alone," one thirty-five-year-old woman named Lucy Lane posted in 2025 on Tik-Tok, "that may have been the only contact they had planned with another person that day, maybe that week." Her post received 98,500 likes.

There's a cost. That ease can become a trap. It can make us forget how much we need in-person interaction. This is what made what happened at Peggy's house so striking. A group of teens woke up early to be together instead of sleeping in. They fought through the friction and inertia to show up in person. And they got something beautiful out of it—the chance to be known and cared for.

Social inertia is real, even among adults. My friend Catherine told me a story about a woman in her life, Lori, who was finding it harder and harder to find motivation to leave the house. Lori started canceling plans at the last minute and then stopped initiating plans with their friend group altogether. Her withdrawal wasn't intentional or mean-spirited. It was just that the pull of staying home to doom-scroll or binge-watch a show on Netflix always seemed stronger than the pull to go out. She kept in touch with friends through texting and social media, and that felt like enough.

Catherine brought it up with Lori when, after multiple attempts to get together, Lori finally agreed to go on a walk. "I wonder if you're giving the best of your attention to your devices," Catherine observed. "What if you saved some of it for people in real life instead?" Lori didn't disagree—she had been feeling the effects of her self-isolation. That night, as she was about to fall into her evening routine of scrolling on her phone and watching Netflix, she dared herself to act. She decided to plan a midwinter party and invited fifteen of her closest girlfriends. To her surprise, every single one RSVP'd yes. But on the day of the party, the texts started rolling in. Eleven friends canceled. Some weren't feeling well, some had childcare issues, and one admitted that she didn't have the energy. When the party hour arrived, only four friends, including Catherine, were seated in Lori's living room. After just an hour and a half, one friend stood up, stretched, and sighed. "I think I'm gonna head home," she said. "I just want to get into my comfy pants and watch TV."

Lori and Catherine suddenly realized that this issue wasn't unique to Lori. This social inertia was *everyone's* problem. As journalist Derek Thompson has noted, "self-imposed solitude might just be the most important social fact of the 21st century." Thompson writes, "The real problem here, the nature of America's social crisis, is that most Americans don't seem to be reacting to the biological cue to spend more time with other people." As we turn to our devices and numb out, we lose the ache that once nudged us toward connection. This kind of isolation doesn't just leave us feeling empty—it also erodes our sense of mattering. When we are at home on our couches alone, we don't get the social proof—like a hand on the arm, a nod, or the warmth of a smile—that shows us we matter to others.

These may seem like small gestures, but they are the building blocks of attunement. When we're together, we're more likely to catch the things people don't say out loud. The Still Face experiment demonstrates how even infants rely on real-time, face-to-face interaction to regulate emotion and build trust. As adults, we may be better at masking our needs, but we still depend on others to see through the mask. And that's much harder to do through a screen. Encouraged by Catherine, Lori started initiating dinners. Friends still cancel occasionally, but her commitment to getting them together has gradually shifted the dynamic in the group. Weeks after Lori began regularly extending invitations, a friend scheduled a birthday dinner for Lori. This time, all but one person came, and they all stayed late. Catherine told me, "I think part of the reason everyone came was because Lori had been so generous with invites and filling other people's mattering cups that they wanted to show up for her." Yes, reaching out requires effort and resistance against the currents of modern life. But the reward is something no screen can offer.

Cut through the static

Just as intertia can hold us back from attuning, so, too, can contending with the tumult of everyday life. After fifteen years of marriage, Emma and John felt more like roommates than partners. Both were thriving professionally, John as a lawyer and Emma as a magazine editor, but home life was more challenging. After the long nightly routine of getting dinner on the table, supervising bath time, reviewing homework, and then tucking the kids in with story time, Emma, exhausted, would relax on the couch to watch TV and get through work emails, while John would retreat to the bedroom to read. They rarely argued, but they also rarely connected. A loneliness had crept into their relationship.

Then one evening, Emma attended a talk about building deeper connections. The speaker shared an exercise called "mental subtraction." "Close your eyes," the speaker instructed. "Now picture an important relationship in your life; maybe it's your partner or a good friend. Picture the day you met them. Next, imagine the ways you might never have met: What if you hadn't gone to that party, taken the bus, or said yes to that blind date? What if this person had never entered your life? Picture the benefits this relationship has given to you over time. Consider how, if you'd never met, you'd have been denied all of them."

Emma's breath caught in her chest. She pictured a world without John, without their wonderful children, and without the home and friendships they'd built together. The speaker's voice broke through her thoughts. "Now, remind yourself that you *did* meet this person. That they're still in your life. Reflect on the good they've brought you—the gifts, both big and small—and let yourself feel grateful."

Tears welled up in Emma's eyes. Driving home that night, Emma felt something shift. Imagining her life without John motivated her to try to find a way to build back the strong relationship they once had. She wanted John to know that she really understood him, but the words didn't come easily anymore. So, instead, the next morning, Emma scribbled a quick note and left it under his coffee mug: "Thank you for always making sure the car is filled with gas. You are such a thoughtful partner." John found the note, and for a second, he stared at it, surprised. Later that morning, he left Emma a note of his own on the kitchen counter: "Thank you for keeping the house running smoothly, even with everything on your plate. I don't know how you do it."

These small gestures of recognition began to soften something between them. Instead of going through their siloed routines, Emma started making bids for attunement. Rather than holding back her stress, she opened up about the worry over a looming deadline. John listened and responded more deeply than in the past. Now, if John noticed Emma looking frazzled in the morning because she needed more time to get ready, he might say, "Why don't I go in late and drop off the kids today? Take the extra time for yourself." As the weeks went by, John and Emma found themselves engaging in new rituals, such as having coffee together before the kids woke up and spending moments on the couch at the end of the day. Slowly, the loneliness in their marriage lifted. In attuning to each other, they were able to find their way back to the connection they thought they'd lost.

As Emma and John learned, the first step toward cultivating attunement is learning to "tune in" to someone else. Think back to old radio dials. Remember how you'd carefully twist the knob to sift through the interference to find the clearest signal? Emotional attunement works the same way. To really connect with someone, you have to cut through the noise, like the distractions of phones, the mental clutter of to-do lists, and the reflex to respond without fully listening. When we learn how to fine-tune our attention, we pick up on the subtle cues of what someone may be feeling beneath the surface. For Emma and John, the static in their relationship came from the whirlwind of their daily lives. It wasn't until Emma took a moment to imagine her life without John, a shock that jolted her into clarity, that she was able to tune in fully again.

Broadcast back

When Greg first became chief, his firefighters felt disconnected from their impact. He also found they suffered from a lack of consistent emotional support. Firefighters pride themselves on being tough, Greg told me, suppressing emotions that they see as obstacles to the job. Vulnerability and asking for help were stigmatized as weaknesses and would often be met with a snarky comment, like "Toughen up, buttercup." To deal with the constant stress, some relied on dark humor, like joking about death, or unhealthy coping mechanisms, like drinking. These attitudes weren't unique to North Charleston. They reflected a broader firefighting culture in which emotional resilience was expected but never openly discussed or supported.

The toll this culture was taking on his firefighters became clear to Greg when he got a phone call from one of his battalion chiefs. A firefighter had been admitted to the psychiatric ward of their local hospital, and he wanted to talk to Greg. Greg dropped what he was doing to meet him. Steve, the firefighter, shuffled out of his hospital room in his pajamas, with his hair uncombed, looking like he hadn't slept in days. Steve explained that years before, he had responded to a call about a young girl who had been shot in the stomach at a drug den. Upon entering the house,

Steve rushed to the girl and applied pressure on her stomach to stop the bleeding and to hold in her intestines. All the way to the hospital, Steve held her and soothed her. When they arrived, doctors and nurses took over. The door to the emergency room closed, and that was it. "After this intense moment, where you're literally holding somebody else's insides, you pass them off to the hospital staff, and you're supposed to just go back to your station and go to sleep—and Steve just couldn't," Greg said.

The next morning, Steve went to the store and bought a stuffed animal like the one his own daughter slept with. He drove to the hospital to give it to the girl, but due to privacy laws, the hospital wouldn't share any information about the young girl. Steve was working overtime, so he had little time to process his experience. The emergency calls he was responding to were relentless, including a stabbing and a fatal accident. The morning after a medical incident involving another young girl, Steve finished his shift, went home, and locked himself in his bedroom. Sensing something was wrong, his wife broke down the door to find Steve with a gun in his hand, planning to shoot himself. This, Steve told Greg, was how he had ended up in the hospital. He had summoned Greg to make a request: "Can you find out if that little girl who was shot in the stomach is alive?"

Greg made some calls and found out that the girl had, indeed, survived because of Steve's heroic efforts. That experience with Steve served as a profound wake-up call for Greg. He resolved never to have something like this happen again to one of his people. "I want them protected and cared for, just as they protect and care for the citizens of North Charleston," Greg said, choking up.

Steve had fallen through the cracks because, like many firefighters, he wouldn't ask for help himself. Tragically, suicide is now the leading cause of firefighter deaths, surpassing those lost in action. Firefighters are help-givers, not help-seekers, Greg explained. They are conditioned to suppress their own needs in service of others, making it all too easy for their struggles to go unnoticed. It wasn't until Steve reached a breaking point that anyone understood how much pain he was in. But Greg understood that the situation wasn't about one man falling through the cracks. It was about a culture blind to the firefighters' need for deeper, more nuanced understanding.

To meet the emotional needs of his firefighters, Greg created a system that was automatic, unavoidable, and preemptive. He began by implementing yearly psychological checkups, a routine one-hour meeting with a clinician, just like an annual physical. It was a structured, judgment-free space to process difficult events. When the calls were particularly difficult, such as ones involving the death of a child, Greg took it a step further and made sure his people were connected with either a chaplain trained in PTSD or a peer counselor who had navigated similar challenges. By showing firefighters that seeking help wasn't a sign of weakness but rather a standard part of maintaining their mental fitness, just like physical fitness drills, Greg hoped to break the stigma.

Greg also wanted to improve the way his team supported one another. To do this, he enrolled his firefighters in Our Community Listens, a three-day course on empathic listening run by the nonprofit Chapman Foundation for Caring Communities. Greg's team learned the skills of attunement, such as how to recognize emotional distress, ask open-ended questions, and listen without immediately jumping to problem-solving mode. The training helped normalize expressing emotions and equipped firefighters with the tools to check in on their colleagues in a way that felt natural rather than forced. By embedding these layers of support, Greg made sure his firefighters would feel heard and understood and not left to carry their burdens alone.

Being heard is so close to being loved that for the average person, they are almost indistinguishable.

—David W. Augsburger

If "tuning in"—genuinely connecting to someone's inner world—is the first step of attunement, then the second step is "broadcasting out," or demonstrating that understanding through meaningful actions. Greg was doing just this with his new initiatives, proactively showing his team that he cared about their inner lives. Attunement is not just about understanding another's inner life but about *responding* in a way that makes the other person feel understood. Instead of saying "You'll be fine" to your nervous child, an attuned response might sound like, "I can see why you're stressed—want to talk it out?" When a nurse recognizes their patient's nervousness, they may offer to hold their patient's hand and spend more time with them. Broadcasting out bridges the internal and external, turning empathy into action and thereby making the internal work of tuning in into a clear expression of mattering. Collectively, Greg's changes embedded attunement into the culture. And the impact is evident in a more open, connected, and emotionally resilient department that values its people as much as the community they serve.

Tune in to yourself

Greg's efforts to broadcast attunement changed his personal relationships, too. One evening, on day two of the listening class, he was sitting on the couch reading when his wife walked into the room to talk about her day. In the past, Greg said, he might have put his finger on his place in the book, signaling that he was only half engaged. But that evening, Greg closed the book and turned his whole body toward his wife to give her his full attention. He listened without distraction. In other words, he was *broadcasting* his attunement to his wife, and she noticed the change immediately. This moment marked a turning point for Greg. Being present and listening showed him how he could be a better husband and father, too.

To truly tune in to another person, we must also, like Greg, be deliberate about tuning in to ourselves. When we're unaware of our emotions, they can easily spill into our interactions. A tough day at work might leave you reacting dismissively to a friend who is opening up because your own mental noise drowns out the moment. Disconnection from our emotions also makes it harder to receive attunement. When someone asks, "What's on your mind?" we may brush them off, unsure how to engage. That's why self-reflection is an important step toward inviting attunement, both in giving and receiving it. By asking yourself questions like "What am I feeling right now? What might be influencing my reactions? What vulnerabilities am I bringing into this moment?," you learn to name your own emotions instead of letting them unconsciously drive your actions. Brain scans show that identifying emotions boosts activity in the brain's emotion-processing center, improving our ability to regulate emotions. When you've tuned in to your own needs and feelings, you're better equipped to step into someone else's inner world with empathy and clarity.

Be an emotion scientist

Tuning in is vital for every kind of relationship. Whether it's with a partner, a child, a colleague, or a friend, the ability to truly listen and connect is what shapes the quality of our interactions and the strength of our bonds. A concept that's helped me with tuning in is to see myself as an "emotion scientist," a term I learned from Marc Brackett at the Yale Center for Emotional Intelligence. Just as scientists seek truth through observation, emotion scientists approach feelings with curiosity, not judgment. They gather clues, like shifts in tone or signs of discomfort, and ask, What might this person be feeling but not saying? By staying open and present to others' emotions, we create a space where they feel safe to share more of themselves, which then opens the door to building a stronger relationship.

> *A real conversation always contains an invitation.*
> *You are inviting another person to reveal herself*

or himself to you, to tell you who they are or what they want.

—David Whyte

We can train ourselves to pick up on these clues, like a slight hesitation before a reply, an overly enthusiastic tone that might be covering nerves, or body language that doesn't quite match someone's words. Responding to these signals with curiosity instead of judgment can open the door to a deeper conversation. I heard a story about a wedding attended by a close group of friends, including one who had just lost her dad. When the bride and her father began to dance, the grieving friend excused herself and headed to the bathroom to collect herself. Without any discussion, the entire group quietly followed her, waiting just outside the bathroom door. When she emerged, they put their arms around her and offered support without saying a word. What a remarkable act of attunement and a testament to how deeply they understood their friend's needs in that moment and how they responded with care.

Feeling like others are attuned to our needs is a hallmark of close, nourishing friendships. In one set of studies, people were asked how well someone close to them, such as a parent, sibling, or friend, really knew them, from their moods and opinions to their personal preferences. What mattered most for relationship satisfaction wasn't how well they *knew* the other person, but whether they *felt known* themselves. That feeling of being seen—really seen—is what deepens connection and creates a sense of support. When it's missing, even strong relationships can start to feel distant. To show this kind of attunement takes a willingness to quiet our own needs long enough to really feel someone else's. You might consider following a tip from journalists, which is to get comfortable with silence and take a moment to respond after someone has finished speaking. When you do this, you create space for more thoughts to surface that might otherwise remain unspoken. Even a simple question, like "How are you *really* doing?" offers us a chance to listen and steady someone when they need it.

Model attunement

Even if you don't yet have people in your life who offer that kind of attunement, you can still take steps to invite it in. Often, when people aren't attuned, it's because they've never been shown how to, or they've learned to turn down the volume on their emotional radar, whether out of self-protection or social conditioning. When you begin to reflect others back to themselves by asking thoughtful questions and deeply listening, you model what attunement looks and feels like and invite others to join you. Not everyone will respond the way you'd like, but even one or two reciprocal connections can begin to make you feel more understood.

> Instead of asking "How are you?," former FBI hostage negotiator Chris Voss offers an observation based on what he sees, such as "You look like you've had a long

> day." This approach, he says, immediately communi-
> cates to people that we are dialed in and aware of their
> needs.

Perhaps the most vulnerable and transformative step in practicing attunement is naming what you need. One woman I interviewed made bids for attunement an inside joke with her friends.
When one was having a rough day, a red flag emoji would be sent
out in the group text, like a flare gun warning to check in. One
red flag generally indicated that someone needed a simple text,
while a double red flag emoji signaled that the sender was going
to need time on the phone to process what had just occurred.

Attunement requires us both to notice that someone is struggling and to intuit what might bring them comfort. Maybe it's a
funny meme or a small act of service, like leaving a favorite snack
on a colleague's desk after a hard day. When someone receives
exactly what they need before they ask, it sends a profound message that they are known and understood. When you lead with
this kind of warmth and openness, you increase the likelihood
that someone will begin to meet you there. And even when they
don't, you're still practicing and becoming more fluent in the language of mattering.

Bridge a divide

You don't need a shared history to practice attunement. In fact,
you can tune in to someone you've never met before. At a political

protest in Austin, Texas, in 2016, Amina Amdeen, a Muslim college student, noticed a young man in a MAGA hat surrounded by an angry crowd. Someone had grabbed his hat. While Amina didn't agree with his politics, she recognized the humiliation and fear in his face because she had felt it, too, the day someone pulled off her hijab in public. Amina stepped forward to defend him and demanded his hat be returned.

That moment of tuning in created a ripple that neither of them expected. Later, in a joint interview, the man, Joseph Weidknecht, said it was the first time he had felt understood by someone he assumed would want nothing to do with him. Amina, too, shared her own experience of feeling different. While they didn't become close friends or change each other's ideologies, attunement allowed them to shift the dynamic in that moment. That's because attunement doesn't hinge on agreement. It rests on the willingness to pay generous attention and to see the person in front of you, even when you don't see the world the same way.

We live in a time marked by division across politics, race, generation, and class. But gaps don't close through argument. They narrow from feeling heard or being seen. When we learn to tune in to a child, a grandparent, or a stranger in a crowd, we practice the kind of attention that can lower defenses and build connection. "I hope that I can be the reason that someone decides to talk to [another person]" said Weidknecht, instead of "cutting them out of their life or blocking them." In an era when algorithms sort us into echo chambers, attunement becomes a bridge and a powerful act of humility and hope.

There's a plate for you

What was most amazing about Grandma Peggy's breakfasts wasn't her willingness to feed ravenous teenagers week after week. It was her ability to create a place for those kids to deeply know one another and to be deeply known, outside of the structure and sometimes restrictive social dynamics of school.

But then, in July 2022, these breakfasts became something more.

Peggy received a devastating phone call. Her grandson, Sam, who'd convinced her to start the Wednesday Breakfast Club, was killed when an oncoming vehicle struck his moped. Peggy's world shattered. "I was completely devastated," she told me.

That very day, his closest friends, regulars at the breakfasts, gathered at Peggy's house to grieve with her. And then, every day that first week, they continued to come by to ensure she was doing okay. "It was hard on me but so hard on them, too," said Peggy. "Losing your best friend at just fifteen must be incredibly hard to comprehend. Not a day goes by that we don't talk about Sam." In the days and weeks following Sam's funeral, Peggy's home remained a space where his friends could gather. When the school year resumed, one asked if the breakfast club would continue. Peggy responded, "If you come, I will feed you."

Instead of dissolving, the Wednesday Breakfast Club grew. More students began showing up, not just Sam's closest friends but others who had heard what Peggy was doing and wanted to be part of it. Some came because they knew Sam; others wanted a place to belong. The club developed a reputation: If you show up at Grandma Peggy's, there's a plate for you.

Continuing to open her home to Sam's friends has helped Peggy cope with her grief and significant health challenges. She has battled cancer multiple times and is living with stage IV colon cancer. Just this year, Peggy lost her daughter, Sam's mother, to a long-term illness. Despite these incredible hardships, Peggy says her Catholic faith and the community she has built around her have kept her strong. As long as she's here, she's determined to take care of her people. "Wednesday breakfasts fill me and keep me going all week," she said.

These days, Peggy feeds thirty or more students every week. News outlets have picked up her story, and when people in St. Louis heard about what she was doing, donations poured in. Neighbors and strangers sent money to help cover the cost of food. Peggy doesn't see it as charity. She believes they just want to be a part of something bigger than themselves. What started as a small favor to her grandson turned into something she could have never imagined, a community that has built itself around grief, comfort, and the simple act of tuning in to each other and showing up week after week. "I think Sam put this breakfast in place so I wouldn't be lonely," she said. She smiled and blinked back tears. "Turns out, he made sure none of us would be."

CHAPTER 6

When the Rug Gets Pulled: Coping with Life's Transitions

I n her best friend's living room, Nancy Schlossberg sat with her hands wrapped around a warm mug of coffee. After twenty years of friendship, Sue's living room was familiar ground, the kind of place where Nancy didn't have to pretend. "My life looks perfect from the outside," Nancy said in a low voice. "So why do I feel so miserable?"

Sue didn't respond right away. She knew Nancy well enough to wait. They'd been talking about how Nancy's recent relocation back to Washington, DC, had thrown her off and how much she missed the structure and routine of her old life. After ten years in Detroit, her husband's role as a union organizer brought them back to Washington when he was appointed general counsel of the United Auto Workers. It felt like the right move. Nancy had landed a prestigious position as the first female executive at the American Council on Education. Her best friend lived across town. Nancy loved Washington. Every box was checked. So why was she feeling so lost?

After listening, Sue suggested that Nancy, a scholar in the field of counseling psychology, turn her analytical mind on herself. "Why don't you make a laundry list of all the factors that shape how people experience change?" she said. "See if you can find patterns." By "factors," Sue meant everything that could influence a transition, such as social support, personal identity, past experiences with change, the amount of control you have over the situation, and even your age or stage of life. This simple prompt energized Nancy. Sue grabbed a pad of paper and a pen, and Nancy began jotting down every variable she could think of: Were there close friends or family nearby? Was the change expected or sudden? Did you choose it, or was it forced on you? Were there financial, emotional, or practical resources that could cushion the landing?

That coffee at Sue's house didn't solve Nancy's disorientation right away. But it gave her a framework to better understand her situation. It helped her see that even the most "successful" transitions come with their own kind of loss. "I was so excited to return to DC, expecting it to be a piece of cake, but what I didn't realize is that even a desired change, if it changes everything, can be upsetting," she told me. Later, Nancy would look back and realize that conversation was the beginning of her life's work studying transitions, both understanding her own and helping others navigate theirs.

Will I ever matter again?

Mattering isn't something we achieve once and then possess indefinitely. Much of our sense of mattering is situational, the value we feel and add in a specific role, like in a fulfilling career, parenting children, or being part of a network of friends who rely on one another. As a result, our mattering can be vulnerable during times of transition, such as Nancy's cross-country move. When the roles and routines that once gave us identity shift, our sense of mattering may begin to slip away. And with that loss of role comes a deeper question: *Will I ever matter this way again?* To carry a sense of mattering through these shifts, we need practices that help us stay anchored in our lives, especially when everything else feels unsteady.

Early in my research, I came across a 1989 academic paper that Nancy wrote about older adults returning to college later in life. Many felt invisible on a campus designed for younger students. Nancy uncovered a striking pattern: that the less students felt they mattered to the college, the more likely they were to drop out. Feeling like you matter, she found, plays a central role in whether people push through transitions or give up. Her findings hit home for me. At the time, my oldest son was getting ready to leave for college, and the word "empty nester" felt too clinical for what I was anticipating. It wasn't just about a quieter house. It was the sense that my most important role—as mother—would shift. When I read Nancy's work, it was as if she had put language to something I hadn't been able to name: that the role

I had inhabited and loved so fully would, inevitably, start to matter less.

This, I realized, is the unnamed pain so many of us face in life's transitions. When the job, the caregiving, or the parenting role no longer fills our days, do we stay anchored to that old identity, hoping to stretch its meaning into the next phase? Or do we need to let go of what was and build something new? Again and again, in the transition stories I kept hearing in my reporting, the answer seemed to be the latter. The challenge wasn't to cling to what was; it was to ask, *Where and how can I matter next?*

Now in her nineties, Nancy was living in a retirement community in Florida when I tracked her down. I left my name and number at the community's front desk, and to my surprise, she called me back the same day. Nancy's warmth and humor and her refreshing openness allowed our conversations to go deep quickly. We discussed the questions that drove her research, like, Who copes well with life's transitions and why? What makes it possible for a person to cope easily with one transition and then struggle with another? Are there ways to help people cope more creatively? In her quest to answer these questions, Nancy researched all kinds of transitions, from geographical relocation to the death of a loved one to divorce. In fact, it was Nancy who developed what's known as "transition theory," a popular framework therapists and counselors use to understand and support individuals experiencing life changes. In her research, Nancy identified three categories of change: "anticipated transitions," or expected changes that occur predictably, such as graduating from school or retiring; "unanticipated transitions," or unexpected changes, such as a sudden job loss; and "nonevent events," or transitions that were expected but did not occur, like the promotion that wasn't awarded or the pregnancy that never happened.

> *Life is in the transitions. We can't ignore these central times of life; we can't wish or will them away. We have to accept them, name them, mark them, share them, and eventually convert them into fuel for remaking our life stories.*
>
> —Bruce Feiler

Transitions are more than logistical changes. They are emotional fault lines. When we lose the roles, relationships, or routines that once reflected our value, it can feel like the ground below us is unsteady. We might start to feel invisible or even unwanted. Nancy's own story of struggling through the relocation back to DC was strangely comforting in that threats to mattering are a universal part of life. No matter how secure we might feel right now, change always comes, and when it does, the roles and relationships that once defined our mattering can shift or disappear. That's the nature of mattering. It isn't an abstract or isolated state that exists in a vacuum. It is necessarily tied to our specific situation. We matter to someone, in something, through a role. We are valued at work, by our friends, as a parent, a partner, or a contributor. So when one of those roles falls away, it's no wonder we start to doubt our worth and our place.

It's not just you

In the midst of a transition, it can be easy to feel like you're alone. Relocating to a new city or being laid off can feel like a solitary challenge. And when we struggle to cope, we might start to believe *we* must be the problem. Our changing circumstances can feel like proof that we are no longer needed or that we're uniquely ill-equipped to cope. Or we might look back on our choices and think we've made a mistake too big to fix. But the fear of inadequacy after a job loss, the grief after the kids leave, the heartache over the divorce—none of this is unique to you. We all struggle to see our worth on the other side of change. You are not alone in this experience, nor are you the problem. As my friend John likes to say, "These feelings are personal but not unique."

The days of a predictable, linear life—one job, relationship, faith, political party, home, and identity—are gone, notes author Bruce Feiler in *Life Is in the Transitions: Mastering Change at Any Age*. Feiler makes the case that people, on average, now go through a disruptive event every twelve to eighteen months. One in ten of these are what Feiler calls "lifequakes," or major transitions. Over half (53 percent) will be out of our control, like losing a job or loved one. The rest of these transitions are of our own choosing, such as getting married or changing careers.

Even exciting transitions can carry an unexpected sense of feeling unmoored. Fresh out of college, Daniel landed his dream job at a fast-growing tech company in Singapore. But when the plane door closed, leaving behind his family and friends hit him hard. He had mattered in so many small ways back home, as the dependable friend you called when you needed help moving or a ride to the airport or advice at two a.m. He always remembered birthdays and showed up early to parties to help set up and stayed late to clean up afterward. In Singapore, that identity fell away. His colleagues were polite but distant. Days went by without meaningful conversation. For weeks, he tried to push through, but the transition remained so painful that he started to feel depressed. Daniel said, "No one warns you that starting over can feel so much like disappearing."

If you're in the midst of a transition and struggling, it can be helpful to remember this: *It's not just you.* That aching sense of not mattering simply proves that you're undergoing something human and difficult. Transitions can make even the most secure person doubt their value. But if others have made it through, so can you. As simple as it sounds, this realization is the first step to reclaiming your mattering. When you understand that others have stood where you are, unsure of their worth or place, and come out on the other side, it becomes easier to believe that you're not stuck here forever, either. A transition is not a terminal state. In fact, it is the opposite. By definition, a transition is the period between one state and another. This liminal space can feel hard, unnerving, and shaky, but as Nancy puts it, "Today is not forever."

When you believe that you're not stuck, you can start to see a way forward. You can get curious. If others have rebuilt their sense of mattering, how can I? That's not to say that any of this is easy. Transitions take a lot of reflection and courage, the kind that doesn't always come naturally. Sometimes you might need to borrow strength from a trusted "cornerman," someone who encourages you to keep going. Sometimes it means finding a good therapist to help you figure out why you're stuck. Transitions, by nature, dismantle the order of things. They interrupt the roles we have held and the plans we had mapped out. They can strip us of the control we once felt, forcing us to pause and confront what's real. Transitions can humble us.

Similarly, we may be pained by seeing our friends and family struggle as they go through their own transitions. And here's a hard truth: You can't build back someone's sense of mattering for them. What you can do is stay close. You can listen, pay attention, and offer steady reminders that they're still needed. Maybe that looks like asking them for advice or asking if they could help a grandchild with homework. Feeling relied on in this way reminds them that they have something important to offer, even when they may not be able to see it for themselves.

A Transition Two-Step

When change hits, here are two steps you can take:

- *First, invite others in.* Let them see and tend to the pain. Seek out stories of others with similar experiences. Read memoirs. Listen to podcasts. Look for meetups with people who are in the midst of the same transition.

- *Second, look outward.* To get out of your own head, go find a need in the world. Remind someone else why *they* matter in small ways—thank the cashier, call your mother, carry a neighbor's groceries, or donate books to a local school. Small acts help rebuild our sense of worth.

Use the mattering lens

Given that none of us is immune to the crashing waves of change, what can we do to sustain and rebuild our mattering through these transitions? How do we keep from losing ourselves when everything around us shifts? If our sense of mattering isn't fixed, how do we learn to matter *for life*? The good news is that there are ways of thinking about our mattering that can equip us for the long haul. Transitions aren't always just losses—if we know what to look for, they can be opportunities to find richer, deeper sources of value and develop a more resilient kind of mattering. Once we stop blaming ourselves for struggling with a transition, we can become curious about what this change reveals about our mattering. We can interrogate our situation more closely.

This is where the mattering lens becomes so powerful. Beyond just the ache of feeling left out or unimportant, the mattering lens invites us to get specific and ask: *What aspect of my mattering has taken a hit?* Am I feeling unseen (a loss of recognition)? Am I missing the feeling that others depend on me (a loss of reliance)? Do I sense that I am not a priority to my boss, my friends, or my family (a loss of importance)? Has my sense of being understood and deeply connected to another been shaken (a loss of attunement)? Do I feel like no one is invested in me—or that I'm not deeply invested in anyone else (a loss of ego extension)?

By pinpointing which facet of our mattering has been disrupted, we can name the deeper need at the root and more thoughtfully consider what will help us rebuild. Maybe you need more acknowledgment at work, or to feel relied on by others, or to be better seen and known by your new community. This understanding offers a clearer view of your situation and a better sense of what to do next.

Every transition is different. Rather than prescribing a one-size-fits-all solution, the mattering lens reveals how each transition challenges us in its unique way and calls for a specific kind of repair. Maybe we need to invest in deeper connections to restore attunement. Maybe we need to try on some new roles to feel relied on once again. Perhaps we need to ask for a turn or set boundaries to renew our sense of importance.

When we develop a habit of checking in with ourselves through the mattering lens—*What aspect of my mattering is feeling threatened right now?*—we become better prepared to anticipate and respond to cracks before they deepen. Over time, this practice builds a deeper understanding of our own mattering needs. Sometimes, the transition itself is clear; perhaps a child leaves for college, a job ends, or a parent dies. But the real loss, the piece of mattering that's missing, is harder to name. What exactly did that role give me? And how do I begin to rebuild that in a different form? The mattering lens helps us stay curious: *What am I really missing? And where can I find it again?*

Using the Mattering Lens: Why am I feeling adrift? Can I name what part of my mattering has taken a hit? My sense of impact? Feeling relied on? Prioritized? Attuned to? Invested in?

Conduct me-search

When researchers decide to pursue a question that holds personal relevance, one that grows out of their own struggles or curiosities, it's somewhat playfully known in academic circles as "me-search." Me-search is the social psychologist who investigates loneliness after grappling with it herself in early adulthood or the developmental researcher who studies resilience in children because he grew up in the foster care system. Rather than a mark against scientific rigor, me-search often leads to more empathetic and nuanced questions, driven by an insider's understanding. For Nancy, me-search was a way of turning her gaze outward, using her own unease ("Why am I struggling with this transition?") as the starting point for curiosity about others ("Why does anyone struggle with a transition, and what helps us move through it?").

Nancy told me about another challenging transition—her

retirement—which coincided with a move to Sarasota with her husband, Steve. On their first Saturday night there, a friend of a friend invited them to a small dinner party. The guests were all in a similar stage of life: a retired architect, a retired dean of a medical school, a retired media interviewer, and the former head of a community foundation. When the former medical dean asked Nancy about her retirement plans, she told him she hoped to work as a consultant to nonprofits in the area. "I am just eager to get involved and see how I can contribute," she said. As she took a bite of the chicken breast, that plan was punctured.

"When I first retired, I thought the same thing," the former medical dean said. "I wanted to help teach a biology course. Not to lead it, just to assist in the teaching of it. But I couldn't get anything." Everyone else at the table confirmed that they had also struggled with finding meaningful ways to contribute to their community postretirement. Nancy's heart raced. These were highly successful people with impressive résumés, and they couldn't land meaningful roles in retirement? This might not just be a temporary difficulty, she thought, but her new, lasting normal.

In Florida, Nancy decided to turn once more to me-search as her compass. She wanted to know who thrives in retirement and why. What attitudes, habits, and support systems make it possible for some people to weather this transition with grace and resilience? To find the answers, Nancy interviewed as many retirees as possible, casting her net wide for stories and insights. She reached out to former professors and administrators at her own retirement community, eager to learn how fellow academics were adjusting to life after work. She interviewed local artists, longtime small-business owners, retired nurses, and even retirees in other parts of the country.

Many people, Nancy found, struggled to feel like they mattered after retiring. Among those she talked to was a former DC police officer who was ready to retire but hadn't given much thought to how he would spend his retirement. He handed in his gun and shook hands with his boss—and that was it. "No one prepared him psychologically," Nancy said. After all those years of being so valued in the community, retirement triggered an identity crisis and a feeling of being irrelevant. The police officer became sullen, withdrawn, and depressed.

At the other end of the spectrum, Nancy found retirees who were, in their own ways, living illustrations of mattering. One woman she met told her that she and her husband had spent almost a lifetime communicating through Post-it Notes. She worked days, and he worked nights, so they connected through scribbled reminders and brief hellos left on the kitchen counter. After retirement, they no longer needed Post-its, because for the first time, they could be truly present to each other, taking walks together, playing cards, and fishing. For the first time in a long time, she felt seen and cherished by her husband. Her mattering came from finally feeling attuned to and prioritized.

Nancy saw that the people who thrived had developed a host of healthy coping strategies. Their stories pointed to what Nancy calls a "recipe for success" for transitions, which includes getting involved and staying engaged, harnessing the power of an invitation, taking initiative, and doing your best to make others feel like they matter. These successful retirees accepted that change is a natural part of life. They maintained an optimistic attitude and relied on social support networks such as friends, family, or colleagues to get them through this transition. They set goals to help maintain motivation and a sense of direction. They also all seemed to recognize that setbacks were temporary and did not define them.

This me-search became Nancy's path back to mattering. She started to apply what she had learned from her interviews to her own life and accepted invitations to join local groups. Bit by bit, these conversations began to lift the feeling of irrelevance. She was not alone. And the exchanges sparked a new direction. Soon she was sharing what she was learning with others, giving talks in the Sarasota area, writing books and articles, and slowly shaping a new identity around her expertise in navigating retirement.

All changes, even the most longed for, have their melancholy; for what we leave behind us is a part of ourselves. We must die to one life before we can enter another.

—Anatole France

Like Nancy, we can all practice me-search after change throws off our sense of mattering. Maybe you turn to books, articles, or research studies related to your experience. Maybe you invite someone who has thrived after a similar transition to tell you their story over coffee. Maybe you seek out workshops and talks to gain practical knowledge. For Nancy, the most transformative knowledge came from reaching out directly to people who'd had similar experiences. In fact, in her interviews, she found that those who coped most effectively often did just this—sought out real-life examples to illuminate their next steps.

Research finds that role models play an important role in supporting psychological well-being and healthy behavior in older adults by helping them overcome limiting beliefs about aging, adopt healthier lifestyles, and stay socially connected. In one study of men aged seventy-five and older, researchers found that role models served as "key sources for behavior change and psychological health benefits" and provided both inspiration and a practical blueprint for how to age.

The great thing about me-search is that it does more than give us strategies for coping. It is also a deeply relational act that strengthens our social ties. When we reach out to learn how someone else has navigated a transition, we send a message that their experience matters to us and that we trust their perspective. In Nancy's me-search, for instance, the retirees she interviewed often told her how meaningful it was to be asked about their stories; they felt seen and appreciated. When we ask others for guidance, we affirm that our role models and their hard-won experience have value. This practice creates an upward spiral of interdependent mattering, where both seeker and sharer feel more connected, valued, and significant.

The act of me-search also empowers us to approach transitions with curiosity. By turning outward, asking questions, seeking stories, and looking for road maps in the lives of others, we shift our perspective from fear of the unknown to an interest in what's possible. Curiosity can help us move beyond our disorientation and consider our next season of life as something of an adventure. Not only does it help us cope better with our immediate change, but it also equips us with the openness we'll need for any transition going forward.

The power of an invitation

Sarah knew the transition back to single life at age forty-five was going to be rough. "How exactly do you function as a single person in a couples' world?" she recalled thinking. Following her divorce, she often felt like an awkward third wheel when socializing with her couple friends. When the check came at dinner and her friends wouldn't allow her to split it, or when the conversation turned to topics like romantic weekends away, Sarah would shrink inside. Instead of feeding her mattering, these dinners made her feel out of place and sometimes even lonelier. Over time, she felt so uncomfortable that she stopped accepting their invitations. During weekends when she had the kids, she chauffeured them around, and when her husband had the kids, she locked herself in her house, drinking more wine than she liked to admit. Her sense of mattering "shriveled up," as she put it.

It faded even more as she pulled away from her friends and kept her struggles to herself. Like many of us, Sarah believed she had to "get her life in order" before reaching out again to her friends. But saying yes doesn't require a perfect life, just a willingness to show up as we are. Researchers call this psychological phenomenon "the beautiful mess effect," or our tendency to overestimate how much others will judge us when we reveal a weakness or failure, while underestimating how much they will appreciate our openness. Studies suggest that while we may see our vulnerability as a flaw, others tend to see it as a strength, a display of warmth, and evidence that we are trustworthy. The very thing we fear might push people away is often what draws them closer. Think of it this way: Have you ever tried to tape something to a slick, shiny surface? It doesn't stick for very long. It's the roughness, the messy part, that gives the tape something to grip. In the same way, it's those imperfect parts of ourselves that create paths to true connection by giving others something real to grasp on to.

Eventually, Sarah and her therapist uncovered the cause of her retreat, a secret fear that her friends were judging or, worse, pitying her. Over time, they developed a strategy focused on reframing her mindset to recognize that invitations were not just about her but about both people in the relationship. In the words of Edith Wharton, "There are two ways of spreading light; to be the candle or the mirror that reflects it." Every yes was an act of giving and a way of helping *others* feel seen and valued. By saying yes, Sarah could be the mirror reflecting their worth.

> In Senegal, a highly regarded value is *teranga*, which emphasizes generosity, openness, and sharing in all encounters, even with strangers. The phrase "thank you" (*jërejëf*) is often followed not by "you're welcome" but by *nio ko bokk*, which roughly translates to "we share it" or "it is for both of us."

Like Sarah, we can shift our thinking to remember that saying yes isn't just for us—it's for the other person, too. Who are the people in your life you can say yes to? How can you accept an invitation you might normally turn down or extend one to someone who might be waiting for it? Perhaps to start, you might set a goal of saying yes or offering an invitation twice in a week. That "yes" helps you when you're feeling lonely, when you're unsure if you matter. And it helps others, too, letting them know that connection with them is worth it. When someone extends an invitation, they're taking a small risk. They're reaching out, making a bid for connection, and hoping we'll meet them halfway. By saying yes, we're accepting that bid and letting them know they matter, too.

When change is bigger than you

It's not just the changes in our personal lives that shake our sense of mattering. Sometimes it's the world itself that shifts beneath us. Large-scale changes can be dramatic and sudden events, such as the COVID-19 pandemic, the attacks on 9/11, or the Global Financial Crisis of 2008, make it immediately clear that the world has shifted. Others unfold gradually over years or even decades, like the erosion of local industries due to offshoring or the encroachment of artificial intelligence into jobs once thought uniquely human. Whether abrupt or slow-burning, these changes remind us that we are living through forces far beyond our control. And in their wake, the roles, relationships, and identities that once gave us a sense of purpose can be stripped away or reshaped beyond recognition, leaving us to question what the future holds and whether we still have a place in it.

Take Sean Butler, a farmer I met who grew up in the 1960s on his family farm in County Roscommon, Ireland, not far from the farm where my grandfather was raised. Sean's farm, passed down through generations, was worked the "traditional way," as he put it. His parents milked a few cows, made their own butter, baked bread, and grew oats, turnips, and potatoes. As a baby, Sean was bundled into a pram and taken to the fields, where farm life imprinted on him from his earliest days. He remembers the peace of lying in the grass as a child, listening to the hum of bees, and knowing he belonged to this patch of earth.

But even during his youth, the "traditional way" of farming was already coming to an end in Ireland. Back then, horsepower from animals was starting to fade, and tractors were just beginning to take over. By age fifteen, Sean was working full-time on the farm and immersing himself in modern farming practices through courses at an agricultural college. He learned that a "good" farmer employed modern methods, such as bulldozing the land and utilizing fertilizer and chemicals to maximize production. Instead of letting cows graze on the grass as his ancestors had, he now gave them feed from the local store to fatten them up faster. The new methods worked. "I was proud of being a farmer," he said. "I felt that farming was a noble thing to do."

As his production picked up, he started noticing changes at home. Sean remembers walking across a field one morning, a day after he had spread slurry (liquid cow manure), and being struck by all the dead slugs and frogs in it. When he had started plowing, he said he wouldn't have gone twenty yards down the field with the tractor before there would be a flock of seagulls and crows following to compete to eat what was being turned up. But by the 1990s, he said, they'd stopped coming because there was nothing to eat. He noticed other changes, too. The wildflowers that were once a fixture in the meadows became scarce. The sound of summertime had been "the corn crake calling," but in the space of a few years, he said, those birds had disappeared. Sean also noticed that the food he was producing wasn't what it used to be. The vegetables often lacked the rich color and taste he remembered from childhood.

As these disturbing observations grew, Sean was also picking up on a change in public discourse that blamed modern agricultural practices for accelerating climate change. He began to feel that farmers were no longer valued for their deep commitment to the land but instead criticized for sowing damage. Connecting the dots between what he witnessed and the messages he heard, Sean began to internalize that guilt and shame. If farming was causing so much damage, he wondered, what did that say about him? "If the crops were unhealthy, if wildlife was being killed, if the effects of all our overproduction were bad, then farming was bad. And if farming was bad," Sean said, "then that meant I was bad." In a fundamental way, he started to feel like a liability.

Just transitions

When the world changes rapidly, people like Sean, and sometimes entire communities, can be left feeling diminished. Their contributions, once essential, become less so, maybe even viewed as obstacles to progress. We've witnessed the human cost of such transformations. In the Pacific Northwest, logging communities began to decline during the early 1980s recession, a downturn that worsened in the 1990s when environmental protections led to widespread mill closures and high unemployment rates. In the 1990s and 2000s, when manufacturing jobs were automated and offshored, millions of jobs were lost, leaving entire regions struggling with economic decline that persists today. In the early to mid 2010s, coal-mining jobs in Appalachia fell dramatically as natural gas became cheaper and environmental regulations tightened, devastating communities where mining had been the economic backbone for generations.

When industries that once provided livelihoods and identities are upended, workers' sense of worth and identity can be shattered. That's because work provides more than income. It provides identity, dignity, and a way of mattering. Economists Anne Case and Angus Deaton have documented how economic displacement contributes to rising "deaths of despair"—suicides, drug overdoses, and alcohol-related deaths—particularly among middle-aged white males without college degrees. One study on suicidal ideation among men found two of the most common words they used to describe their pain were "useless" and "worthless."

As we look to the years ahead, the stakes of not mattering are rising fast. Economists at Goldman Sachs estimate that artificial intelligence (AI) could automate or impact as many as 300 million jobs globally. The pace of this transformation is unprecedented. Technology leaders like Bill Gates predict that within the next decade, advances in artificial intelligence could make humans unnecessary for many of the tasks we do today. "It's very profound and even a little bit scary—because it's happening very quickly, and there is no upper bound," Gates has said. With automation and AI threatening to displace millions of jobs, some experts have proposed universal basic income (UBI) as a solution to provide economic security. While UBI trials have shown promise in reducing poverty and improving mental health, income alone cannot replace the psychological benefits of meaningful work.

When machines take over tasks that once gave people identity and purpose, our need to feel valued and to add value won't fade. If anything, it will grow more urgent. The concept of a "just transition" offers a starting point for how to meet this challenge. First introduced by labor unions decades ago to protect workers affected by environmental regulations, just-transition policies, such as retraining, job placement, and investing in impacted local economies, aim to ensure that the costs of change don't fall hardest on the most vulnerable communities. In the age of AI, we need to expand on the idea of just transitions to reimagine how people can feel valued and add value as machines take on more cognitive and creative tasks.

In shaping the future of work, the central question can no longer be limited to *What will people do?* We must also ask, *How will people know they matter?* The answer requires a policy framework rooted in the principles of mattering. That means designing systems that both safeguard economic security and also uphold human dignity, ensure social connection, and promote a sense of meaningful contribution. If we are to build a resilient and inclusive future, every person must be able to see themselves as an essential and valued part of the world taking shape around them.

Update your title

A few years ago, Nancy received a call from Erin McLeod, the CEO of Senior Friendship Centers in Florida. By then, Nancy's work on retirement and transitions had made her somewhat of a local celebrity. Erin explained that the center hoped to launch a small group for older adults to create a space for people who wanted to talk candidly about the challenges and opportunities of aging. Erin hoped Nancy could facilitate the group together with Michael Karp, a former lawyer with a gift for getting people to talk. Nancy agreed immediately, and in their first planning session, she, Michael, and Erin worked out the group's purpose, which was to bring together retirees in their seventies, eighties, and nineties every Tuesday to discuss the issues that define the last third of life, such as how to cope and stay resilient with the big and small losses that can come with aging.

While Nancy and Michael would guide the discussions, they saw themselves as students as much as leaders, ready to learn from others' wisdom, and hoped to create a community where all the members of the group would support one another. The final item on the agenda for the planning session was to create a name for the group. They tossed around ideas until Erin, with a grin, suggested "Aging Rebels." The group broke into laughter, and in unison, Nancy and Michael agreed: "That's it."

During one of my Zooms with Nancy, she invited me to Sarasota to sit in on one of the Aging Rebels' meetings. Inside the center, seniors sat at tables taking classes and playing cards in the light-filled common room. Nancy and I made our way into the library, where the Aging Rebels meet each week. One by one, people trickled in. Nancy greeted each person with a hug and offered me a personalized introduction: "Janet is always the first to arrive," and "Sarah is such a good listener." To another woman, Nancy said, "You always look so elegant." And always one to squeeze in a joke, Nancy added, "But you know, my eyesight isn't so great anymore."

At the start of the meeting, Nancy asked members to share any of the group's past conversations that had really stuck with them. One retiree recalled a lively discussion about business cards. How do you describe yourself to the world when you no longer have a job to lean on? One former journalist had updated his card, swapping out his profession for "Concerned Citizen." It was a conscious shift to reflect what mattered most to him now, namely, being engaged in his community rather than holding on to a title. Someone else mentioned a friend who'd made up cards that read, "Retired. Ask someone else." Everyone laughed.

Nodding along, Nancy opened up about her own business cards. At the University of Maryland, where she was a professor and the head of a human resources center, her business card was crowded with type, signifying that she was *somebody*. After she moved to Florida, all those words became null and void. She went to a local stationery store to get cards printed with just her name and email to hand out to new people she met. She felt like "a nobody," she said, and the blankness of the cards reinforced that feeling. Finally, after finding purpose through her retirement research, she printed new cards. These cards were bright red, with her name in white on one side and "Author. Speaker. Consultant" on the other. Nancy said, "My business card went from a lot of words to nothing to finally a bright red card that felt like me."

Redefining our roles

Reclaiming our mattering doesn't have to mean rewriting our entire business card. Sometimes, our title stays the same, and what changes is the meaning we give to it. Rather than completely reinventing ourselves, we can redefine the roles we already have. Think of a parent whose children have grown and left home. Their title, parent, doesn't end. It's the job description that has changed. We can fortify our mattering by reimagining that role.

This was the case for Sean Butler. The despair he felt over the damage his farm was inflicting—on the land, environment, animals, crops—made him question his title of farmer. Rather than give up, he learned how to hold on to the title by redefining the role. At first, he thought the answer might be organic farming. In 2001, he gradually weaned his fields off chemical inputs, and slowly, he saw some glimmers of hope. His food quality improved; his cattle required fewer antibiotics. But organic farming did not entirely support the natural processes of the land; it mostly focused on removing chemicals. The approach didn't make his land worse, but it also didn't necessarily make it better.

Sean wondered what more he could do. In 2021, thanks to the

documentary *Kiss the Ground*, he discovered a concept he'd never heard of, called regenerative farming. This, he felt, was what he'd been searching for all his life. He learned everything he could. He began to manage his land in a way that promotes the health of the soil microbiome, which includes bacteria, fungi, and other microscopic life, and changed his grazing practices, moving his animals from area to area every day so that the grass could grow longer. The animals would eat only about half of the grass in a certain area, while the other half would be trampled down and serve as food for the soil. The healthier soil led to faster recovery of the land, and Sean noticed a gradual increase in biodiversity on his farm. Skylarks, flowers, orchids, dung beetles, bees, ladybirds, and other insects returned. Now he is producing as much food as he did before, but it is more nutrient-dense and tastes better.

His new practices also help reduce air pollution, water pollution, and water runoff. "There are very few things in the whole climate change problem that cannot be helped by farming regeneratively," he told me. He spoke to me with energy and passion, a stark contrast to the disillusionment he once felt. The government had taken notice, too, offering grants to replant all the trees that were bulldozed in the 1950s and 1960s. Sean is now busy sharing what he knows with other Irish farmers who are feeling lost. Although the European Union had been imposing new environmental policies, these regulations often lacked sufficient guidance and support. Sean's experience gives us a glimpse of what a just transition can look like, not by just imposing change but by working alongside those most affected to create sustainable solutions. Rather than being cast aside, farmers like Sean can be invited to be part of the solution.

For Sean, his reinvention as a regenerative farmer has given him a renewed sense of his value to his community. His quest to make sense of his crisis—his me-search—helped him move beyond the narrow boundaries of his former identity and get curious about a future of stewardship and innovation that benefits both him and others. Sean now opens his farm once a week to something called "social farming," in which people with special needs come out to the farm and contribute their work for a few hours. "I've always known that nature is a great healer," said Sean, "but to see what a difference it can make for someone to move cattle, put up a fence, cut a bit of timber—I'm told it's transformative." He loves that the experience helps others, even as they are helping him. "I used to see the farm as something that I owned," he said. "Now I see that I belong to the land. I've found my part in that symbiotic relationship, where I can contribute to the whole web of life. It feels a bit like coming home."

After the Aging Rebels meeting, Nancy invited me back to her condo, a sunny space with a view of the Sarasota Bay. She opened a drawer in her desk and pulled out a neat stack of business cards, some vibrant red. As she thumbed through them, Nancy reflected on how far she'd come since moving to Florida. She'd built an entirely new sense of purpose through her research on retirement and her work with the Aging Rebels. The group has drawn the attention of graduate students from the University of South Florida who are studying aging, a full-circle moment for a scholar who spent her career examining transitions. "This group is very rewarding," she said. "My life is as good as it could be."

Nancy tucked the cards back into the drawer and then looked up with a smile. "And now I have no card," she said. "I'm beyond the evolution of business cards." At first, I was puzzled—just moments earlier, she showed off the red cards as a symbol of her new identity. But as we continued to talk, I understood. The cards had been a way to steady herself through transitions and placeholders until something deeper took root. With her mattering now well established in this new phase of her life, Nancy no longer needed a title to define her worth. It lived in her relationships, in the community she helped build, and in the meaning she created on her own terms.

"Do you feel like you matter now, Nancy?" I asked her.

Nancy leaned back on her chair, smiled, and said, "I would say unequivocally, yes, I matter. I truly feel I matter."

CHAPTER 7

How We Spend Our Days: Mattering at Work

When Nancy Schlossberg talked to me about retirement, she spoke about how difficult it was to cope with the sudden absence of structure, identity, and sense of being needed that work provided. But many of the people I interviewed felt the opposite. They weren't dreading retirement—they were desperate for it. The real crisis wasn't looming in the distance. It was already unfolding at work, where a slow erosion of mattering had left them feeling invisible and expendable.

Frankie, a remote worker in education sales, told me that at work she felt like a "hologram" flattened into "a quota-chasing widget," not a full human worthy of being known by her boss and colleagues. Victoria, a physician, complained that she was forced to dedicate more time to completing patient forms on a computer than interacting with her real patients. "It feels like death by a thousand clicks," she said, talking about the burnout she was experiencing. John, an investment banker, confided that he had barely slept the night before our interview after being deliberately excluded from the final decision on a deal he'd worked on for over a year. As I listened to these stories, I thought of that Annie Dillard line: "How we spend our days is, of course, how we spend our lives." If most of our days are spent at work, and we don't feel like we matter there, then how can we feel like we matter in our lives?

When we talk about the global epidemic of burnout, disengagement, or quiet quitting, we are naming the surface-level symptoms. At their root is a deeper crisis of mattering. Workers no longer feel valued, and too often the value they add goes unrecognized. The numbers tell the story. In 2024, US employee engagement, measured as "the involvement and enthusiasm" of employees in their work and workplace, fell to 31 percent, its lowest in a decade, echoing a global decline in workforce engagement over the past five years. Two-thirds of employees worldwide report either "struggling" or "suffering," with only one in three considered truly thriving, according to Gallup. The most common description among disengaged employees I interviewed was that they "felt like a cog in the machine."

What we are witnessing is the predictable outcome of systems that have forgotten to treat people as people, argues Irish social entrepreneur Dale Whelehan. He writes, "We've built entire systems on the assumption that humans are machines. Replaceable. Optimizable. Unemotional. Always on. And now, we're cracking." Setting aside the human toll, the financial cost of this crisis is staggering. Disengaged employees are more likely to leave, and replacing those employees is expensive. Gallup estimates that leaders and managers cost around 200 percent of their salary to replace, while employees in technical roles cost 80 percent and frontline workers cost 40 percent of their salary. What's particularly disheartening is that much of employee turnover can be preventable. Gallup found that employees who felt authentically and personally recognized were 45 percent less likely to have changed organizations two years later. Even the least human-centered corporation is well incentivized to address this crisis.

The rapid adoption of generative AI is intensifying the sense of replaceability among workers. In a *Wall Street Journal* article titled "'Everybody's Replaceable': The New Ways Bosses Talk About Workers," Shopify CEO Tobi Lütke warned that his company won't make new hires unless managers can prove AI isn't capable of doing the job. The same article quotes a staff memo from Micha Kaufman, CEO of the freelance marketplace Fiverr, saying, "AI is coming for your jobs. Heck, it's coming for my job too. This is a wake-up call." He adds that those "who will not wake up and understand the new reality fast are, unfortunately, doomed."

Leaders themselves aren't immune to workplace burnout. A 2025 leadership survey revealed a troubling trend, noting that 71 percent of leaders reported a substantial increase in stress since assuming their current roles. Among those leaders who reported heightened stress, over half (54 percent) expressed fear of burnout, and 40 percent admitted they had considered stepping away from leadership altogether.

Seeing these warning signs, many organizations are working harder than ever to stem the tide, rolling out programs designed to combat burnout and boost morale, only to watch engagement scores continue to plummet. When leaders are overwhelmed and teams are disengaged, the instinct is often to reach for familiar tools, such as bringing in a consultant, conducting a survey, or scheduling leadership training. These aren't bad solutions. Surveys can identify areas to improve, and leadership training can prompt self-reflection and skill building that leads to better management. But too often, these programs address the symptoms, not the source, and become replacements for deeper, more sustaining repair. The language we use around these solutions reveals the problem. When companies talk about "empowering employees" or "building resilience," they shift the burden back onto people already overwhelmed by the system. These approaches signal that we'd prefer to teach people how to cope with not mattering rather than change the conditions that leave them feeling like they don't.

As part of my research, I conducted an international survey of over two thousand employees across industries, which was administered by Centiment between February and April 2024. I asked respondents to recall specific moments when they felt they didn't matter at work and moments when they did.

Anti-Mattering Moments:	Mattering Moments:
• "When my ideas were dismissed, I felt unheard and underappreciated." • "I just don't feel anything I do is praised." • "When I was injured at work, they did not show concern." • "Whenever [my] manager [is] rude to me." • "When my parents died within four weeks of each other, my boss sent me a very nasty email. I was shocked." • "Most days [I don't feel like I matter]."	• "When my boss asked for my opinion." • "When my boss praised my work on a challenging project, I felt valued and motivated to continue contributing to the team's success." • "When a colleague said, 'I love working with you.'" • "My manager sent me a Christmas card thanking me for all I do and the kindness I have shown her." • "When I was shown leniency." • "Every day [I feel like I matter], as they are always saying, 'thanks' and 'good work.'"

The business case for mattering

In my research on the power of mattering at work, I traveled across the country, visiting organizations that were defying the trend, where employee engagement and well-being were high. My research took me to visit one hotel chain where housekeepers, breakfast attendants, and the person who handles customer complaints—people in often thankless roles—loved their jobs so much that they stayed for decades. At a factory in Wisconsin, I saw something I didn't expect: workers tearing up as they described feeling so cared for at work that they went home energized and able to be better, more present partners and parents. I met with attorneys in large law firms, finance executives, medical staff at busy hospitals, employees at nonprofits, and educators who, despite the pressures inherent in their professions, were thriving. I interviewed CEOs, managers, and frontline workers; sat in on team meetings; and read through hundreds of workplace surveys.

What I found was striking. No matter the industry, size, or structure, these organizations had arrived at the same fundamental truth. That is, when employees know they matter, they work harder, stay more loyal, and bring more passion to their roles. Put another way, treating employees like they matter is not just the right thing to do—it's also good business. These organizations were guided by the principles of mattering and made sure their employees knew that they were valued, that their work had an impact, and that their roles were essential to the company's success and to the people around them.

As I spent time in these workplaces, I kept coming back to a metaphor: fuel. Modern workplaces, I came to see, run on one of two kinds—clean or dirty. Dirty fuel uses fear and hypercompetition to motivate. It's a workplace where trust and appreciation are rare. Dirty fuel might drive short-term results, but it slowly corrodes the engine, leaving employees fatigued, cynical, and disengaged. By contrast, the "mattering" workplaces I visited ran on clean fuel. Here, best intentions were assumed, contributions were seen, and people felt connected to a purpose larger than themselves. Clean fuel motivates and energizes people to give more because they want to.

Still, what I've come to realize is that switching fuels isn't enough. The dirty fuel must be flushed out. Anti-mattering—the subtle and overt ways people are made to feel invisible, unvalued, or replaceable—is sludge in the system, eroding workplace culture. When researchers study "anti-mattering," they ask questions like "How often have you been treated in a way that makes you feel like you are insignificant? To what extent have you been made to feel like you are invisible? How much do you feel like you will never matter to certain people? How often have you been made to feel by someone that they don't care what you think or what you have to say?"

In the workplace, anti-mattering can show up in big ways, like racism, discrimination, or firing people in an uncivil manner, without warning, by locking them out of their laptops or deactivating their key cards. More often, it shows up in more subtle ways, like dismissiveness, a chronic lack of acknowledgment, or rudeness. When we're met with rudeness, we receive a signal to our brains that we aren't valued. And when our sense of mattering is threatened, it hijacks our focus. Instead of staying present with the task at hand, our attention shifts to replaying the interaction, trying to make sense of the slight. The mental energy we'd normally devote to our work gets consumed by the effort to reestablish our sense of worth. In one role-playing experiment, medical teams were exposed to either neutral treatment or rudeness by an "expert" who suggested that they "wouldn't last a week" in his department. In the aftermath, researchers found the team exposed to rudeness offered the wrong diagnosis, resuscitated or ventilated inappropriately, communicated poorly, prescribed the wrong medications, and made other egregious errors. Antimattering impacts decision-making and disrupts performance.

Some leaders might dismiss the idea of investing in a culture of mattering as a luxury, but the evidence suggests organizations can't afford not to. Gallup finds that when employees strongly agree that their organization cares about their overall well-being, they're four times more likely to be engaged, 53 percent less likely to be actively job hunting, and seven times more likely to recommend their workplace as a great place to work. They are also 73 percent less likely to feel burned out and 50 percent more likely to be thriving in life. It also translates directly to business results. Gallup found that highly engaged teams are 23 percent more profitable than their disengaged counterparts, thanks to stronger performance, sharper awareness of customer needs, and tighter-knit collaboration.

Data from Great Place to Work provides even more compelling evidence. The Fortune 100 Best Companies to Work For, as voted on by their employees, have outperformed the S&P 500 over the past twenty-eight years, especially during economic downturns. When a crisis occurs—think the dot-com crash—the 100 Best Companies double the gap between themselves and the S&P 500. Simply put, when organizations invest in a culture of mattering where people feel valued and depended upon, performance and retention improve.

So, what does it look like to *lead* with mattering in the workplace? First, we must recognize that the demands on today's leaders are unprecedented. They're managing hybrid teams, navigating economic uncertainty, implementing new technologies, and trying to hit increasingly ambitious targets. They didn't create the systems that got us here, and they're likely doing their best within the constraints they inherited. If you are a manager feeling overwhelmed by yet another item to add to your to-do list, let me reassure you: Mattering isn't one more thing to put on that list. It's a new lens through which you can view your responsibilities, from structuring meetings to celebrating wins to handling failures. Importantly, the mattering lens helps you identify and address issues before they worsen.

When we hear the word "leadership," we often picture someone in a management position. But creating a culture of mattering relies on the efforts of every single employee. A leader can be the partner at a law firm as well as the receptionist, who has the critical role of making everyone feel welcome and keeps the workplace organized and functioning efficiently. A leader might be a junior member of the team who recognizes the investment in them by a senior staff member. Or it could be a colleague who consistently extends trust to their coworkers. Similarly, these ideas belong in every type of workplace: hospitals, schools, commercial kitchens, construction sites, retail shops, factory floors, loading docks, law enforcement, and behind the wheel of a delivery truck. So if you're in a supporting role or just embarking on your career and wondering whether mattering leadership applies to you, it does. Mattering is about bringing an awareness to the small, everyday moments that either affirm a coworker's value or erode it. And it's in those small moments, multiplied over time, that all of us can shape a workplace culture.

The Mattering Core at Work

Principle	For Yourself	For Your Colleagues
Recognition	Keep an "impact file" to track your contributions.	Call out specific wins or strengths. Let people know how their work made a difference.
Reliance	Notice when others count on you.	Give someone a meaningful responsibility. Let them know you trust them to deliver.

Importance	Set boundaries that protect your time and well-being because you are a priority.	Check in on a coworker's well-being during a stressful time. Be clear that you value your colleagues as people, not just workers.
Ego Extension	Surround yourself with people who root for your success.	Be the person who champions someone else's growth. Celebrate their wins as your own.
Attunement	Notice your emotions, energy levels, and stress responses, and respond with care.	Personalize your support by listening and responding to what's not being said.

Connect colleagues with their impact

When I arrived at the factory of BW Papersystems in Phillips, Wisconsin, it was buzzing with activity. Men and women were assembling machines that make corrugated cardboard boxes. As I toured the floor, something drew my attention. I noticed a card displayed next to each machine. One manager smiled when I asked him about them. "Ah, those are story cards," he said. He explained that the company started creating these cards when leaders realized something was missing on the factory floor—the sense of who the job was ultimately for. Projects arrived in code, as strings of letters and numbers like 4K152 and 7G311. Workers rarely knew where their machines would end up or who would use them.

Imagine getting to your workstation each morning greeted only by the label "7G311." Would you feel inspired to do your best work? Or know why it was significant? It's easy to see how you could feel like a cog in a machine. Instead, these "story cards" show how each piece fits into the final product, with a photo and a story about the person who would one day use it. The story cards show employees exactly how their contributions matter within and beyond the organization, giving their work new meaning.

Connecting employees with their impact can take many forms. It might look like an office manager who gathers stories from satisfied customers and shares them with the team. Or a shift supervisor who posts photos of where finished products end up. Or it might start with sticky notes, like it did at a nonprofit I visited.

For years, the doors of the social workers' offices at a New York City nonprofit were filled with Post-it Notes from people the organization served; each one was scribbled with a message of gratitude. "Thank you for listening when no one else would." "You saved my family." But just down the hall, the doors in the accounting and development offices were bare. These employees sat behind computer monitors and spreadsheets, doing the invisible but critical work of keeping the programs funded. Leadership noticed the gap in recognition. So one Monday morning, the executive director tacked up a sign in the entryway of the office: *Wall of Appreciation. Tell someone they made a difference.* Below the sign was a stack of index cards, pushpins, and a jar of pens. The executive director started by posting a note of thanks to her assistant. "Becky, thank you for keeping this organization running smoothly. Without your organizational skills, we'd be so much less effective."

Pretty quickly, more cards appeared. "Thanks to Mark in accounting for finding the money we needed to keep that family in their apartment." "Development team, because of your efforts, hundreds of young people will have winter coats this year. Thank you." With its pushpins and index cards, the bulletin board transformed into a mirror, reflecting the significance of each employee's efforts. These weren't vague thank-yous. They were specific about each person's unique impact on the organization. The change was palpable, the executive director told me. Morale lifted. People who once stayed quiet in meetings began speaking up, offering ideas and asking questions. They felt seen. Significant. Depended on. "It's the first time the back office has truly felt like part of the mission," she told me.

> *Far and away the best prize that life offers is the chance to work hard at work worth doing.*
>
> —Theodore Roosevelt

You don't need to be in a leadership role to help a colleague bridge the gap between what they do and the positive impact of their actions. When people experience firsthand how their work improves the lives of others, they gain a deeper sense of purpose and pride in what they do. (Think of Greg and his firefighters in South Charleston.) Wharton professor Adam Grant has found that even brief face-to-face contact with the people who benefit from our work—customers, clients, patients, or students—can significantly boost motivation across professions, from engineers and nurses to call center reps. In one study, university fundraisers who spent just five minutes speaking with scholarship recipients raised twice as much money as those who didn't. Having a direct connection to your impact increases motivation and resilience.

Rely on them

One of the most telling signs of a struggling workplace is when people stop trusting and relying on each other. Reliance means feeling depended on *and* trusted to come through. Trust signals confidence. It's another way of telling someone they're valued. But in toxic workplaces, trust erodes. Employees tend to second-guess each other. They might hoard tasks, operate in silos, and then stop depending on one another altogether. This was Joelle Salerno's experience. For three years, she worked in an office rife with mistrust and suspicion. Bosses assumed the worst intentions. Employees couldn't do their best work because they were too preoccupied with office politics and avoiding blame or public humiliation. Eventually, she decided she'd had enough. When she walked into an interview with Chad Jones, executive director of the Electrical Contractors Association of Western Pennsylvania, she was looking for more than a new job. She was looking for a healthier workplace.

The first surprise of the interview came when Chad told Joelle, "I don't need you in the office nine to five—I just need you to do the work." She couldn't help but be suspicious. What kind of boss wouldn't want their employees in the office so they could surveil their every move? But Chad meant it. Then came another surprise. Chad explained that he would be hiring her to fill a new government affairs role, but he didn't pretend to know better than she what that position should look like. Instead, he wanted her to build out the role herself since she was the one with the government experience. It was something Joelle had never experienced at work before. "The idea that someone could just . . . trust me?" she told me. "This can't be real."

When your manager hands over an important project, they're saying, *I trust your judgment.* When a colleague encourages the team to weigh in on how tasks should be divided, or a supervisor asks for input on improving daily operations, they're signaling that employees are trusted to help shape the workplace in meaningful ways. Motivated by Chad's trust, Joelle extends that same trust to the people she works with. Outside of her day job, she leads a summer program for girls interested in construction careers. It introduces teenagers to trades like welding, carpentry, and electrical work. Joelle is the director, but she doesn't micromanage those she works with. When a team of professional bricklayers volunteered to run a session at the camp for the first time, their lead turned to Joelle and asked what kind of activities they should plan for the girls. Joelle simply said, "You know this work best. I trust you." That trust allowed the bricklayers to get creative. They set up hands-on stations for tile setting, stonework, and tuck-pointing. The session was a hit. The girls jumped in, excited to try something new.

> In the famous Hawthorne Studies at Western Electric, researchers discovered that involving workers in choices about something as basic as their workspace lighting boosted morale and productivity. They found that when the lighting improved, output increased, but also, when they decreased the lighting, the output increased further. Researchers concluded that it wasn't the lighting itself that affected the workers but the feeling that they mattered, that they were of special interest rather than being anonymous and unrecognized workers, which spurred productivity.

In my interviews, I was struck by how often being trusted and relied on inspired others to adopt the same leadership approach. Another example was Jason Schumacher, a customer care manager at Trek Bikes. In 2018, he was stunned when he received the results of his team's Great Place to Work employee survey. The score of 64 wasn't catastrophic, but it was a steep drop from previous years, and the feedback, which ranked his communication low, completely blindsided him. Reading the survey results aloud in front of his team was so hard for Jason that he had to step out of the room to collect himself.

When he met with his boss, Laurie Koch, Trek's VP of global customer service, to review the survey, she didn't treat the score as a reflection of Jason's failure. She didn't demand oversight into how he'd fix it. Jason said that she simply listened to him, validated how hard it felt, and communicated her confidence that he would find a way to address his team's complaints and improve the score.

Deciding to follow Laurie's example, Jason entrusted his team with helping him find solutions. He adopted a practice he learned from Laurie, in which employees could write her a "Dear Laurie" letter that outlined a concern and a potential solution to the problem. Jason proposed a "Dear Schumacher" letter, encouraging his team to meet without him to discuss their concerns as a group, write their letter, and share ownership of the proposed solutions. He also started a daily team huddle in which he rotated leadership of the meeting so everyone had a chance to share responsibility for the agenda. By transferring ownership of the meetings, Jason made his colleagues feel trusted enough to share constructive feedback and to shape their workplace into a more supportive environment. This approach rewards trust with more trust and tangible results. In 2019, just one year later, Jason's team's Great Place to Work score jumped from 64 to 94.

Prioritize well-being

Katherine felt the stress in her shoulders first, the tightness that developed from too many hours hunched over her laptop trying to meet an unrealistic deadline. Her remote team was working on a climate change report that synthesized years of research across three continents and that had been dropped on her team's desk mere weeks before it was due to be published. It required late-night calls with partners in Asia and early-morning edits for European stakeholders. The work was intense and made harder by the absence of real leadership. Their manager rarely checked in, and when she did, she offered vague, impersonal feedback. No one was asking how members of the team were holding up. No one seemed to care. The only thing that seemed to matter was the deadline.

But in those high-pressured days, something else happened. Katherine's teammate Raj started sending end-of-day messages, like "Hope you'll log off soon—you've done enough today." Another colleague, Eva, began scheduling short afternoon breaks where they'd jump on Zoom for quick "check-ins." Katherine reciprocated by stepping in when a colleague seemed stretched too thin: "Want me to take that section off your plate?" Even as they neared the deadline and the stress intensified, they continued to look out for one another, pointing out each other's good work, asking about a family member who had just had surgery, and reminding each other that they were worthy of breaks. In a workplace that didn't seem to care about the toll the project was taking on its employees, this team created a buffer for one another. For that grueling month, they became stewards of each other's mattering.

What they were building, without knowing it, was something similar to what researchers have termed "Fast Friends," an evidence-based exercise that helps build trust, connection, and well-being in adult friendships and workplace teams. In that exercise, participants take turns responding to increasingly meaningful prompts that foster the kind of emotional openness that deepens bonds. For example, one prompt is, "Before making a telephone call, do you ever rehearse what you are going to say? Why?" Another prompt is, "What would constitute a 'perfect' day for you?" Although Raj, Eva, and Katherine did not use a formal list of questions, they instinctively took turns opening up and caring for each other by sharing encouragement, checking in, and offering help, which created the same effect. In a workplace that failed to see them, this care made them visible to one another. As Katherine discovered, protecting mattering in the workplace doesn't have to start with management. Sometimes, the most meaningful kind of leadership comes from the person sitting next to us.

Even small, consistent gestures of care can create an outsized impact. Companies that prioritize employees, whether through flexible work policies, robust mental health support, or ensuring fair workloads, see significantly lower turnover and absenteeism. Frankie's story exemplifies this. After leaving a teaching career she loved because of a chronic illness, Frankie pivoted into a role in literacy curriculum sales. The position was remote, which was ideal given her health needs. But almost immediately, red flags emerged. "There was constant micromanagement," she said. "You had to be in nonstop communication, and they tracked how often our computers were active." The constant surveillance was demoralizing and distracted her from the work itself.

After several months, she began scanning job boards. When a job opened at a state agency, she took it—even though it meant a pay cut and the added structure of three in-office days each week. Her new employer offers flexibility with work-from-home days, flextime, and the understanding that its employees are people with personal demands and lives outside the office. A year after taking the job, Frankie is thriving. "No one's watching my every move. My work speaks for itself. If I have a doctor's appointment or need to take the dog to the vet, I don't have to lie or put in a request for a personal day two weeks ahead of time that might get denied anyway. Now, I just say I'll be back in an hour, and no one questions me." The ironic thing, Frankie said, is that even though the curriculum sales position was fully remote, it felt less flexible and less oriented toward employee well-being than her current job, where she has autonomy to do her work *and* take care of important personal needs. When I asked if this workplace made her more productive and more engaged at work, Frankie didn't hesitate. "Absolutely," she said. "I want to do well so I can stay in this job forever."

Personalize support

Scott was shaking so hard he could barely hold his vision board. It was the last day of leadership training at the headquarters of Jersey Mike's, a national sandwich chain, and each member of the twenty-person class was expected to present their board. The young manager had pulled the director of training and development, John Hughes, aside before the presentations began. "I have an anxiety disorder," he whispered. "There's no way I can do this." Hughes answered, "That's okay. You don't have to present, but if that changes, we'll be here."

This kind of exchange is not unusual in Hughes's training rooms. I'd heard about the training from my husband, Peter, who sits on the board of Jersey Mike's. Many participants are under twenty-five and often new to leadership. Over the past several years, Hughes has expanded the training into a human-centered program that, along with management skills, also emphasizes personal growth. Hughes—affectionately known as "Coach Hughes"— and his small team sit with participants at lunch, get to know their individual learning styles, and create a space where people feel heard and individually supported. By the end of the training, something remarkable often happens. The same people who entered the room unsure of their place in the company would end up standing before their peers and opening up about where they've come from and what they hope to accomplish.

In this case, Scott stood up after all. As he struggled through the first few lines of his story, his classmates began calling out, "You got this. We're here." A few walked over and stood beside him in solidarity. One put his hand on his back. Scott made it through. And when he did, the room burst into applause. Hughes calls these moments the "epiphany of the week"—not just that someone can stand and speak, but that they've been given the emotional scaffolding to do so.

After forty years at the company, Hughes recognizes that offering attunement enables people to do their best work, creates stronger teams, improves company results, and develops people into the leaders they want to be. Leaders and coworkers who tune in to the inner lives of their employees sense when a team is out of sync, when someone's voice isn't heard, or when they just need a little more support.

Attunement is foundational for organizational success. We tend to think of navigating emotions in the workplace as a "soft" skill, but it's actually a life skill that yields concrete results. Managers with high emotional intelligence have teams that are 20 percent more productive than those with low EQ, measure 34 percent better in team problem-solving effectiveness, and show 27 percent higher performance ratings and 40 percent higher employee retention.

It was this kind of leadership that shaped Jake Huskey. Jake is a site operations director responsible for 220 team members at Barry-Wehmiller's packaging equipment facility in Duncan, South Carolina. (He works within the same company that owns the BW Papersystems plant.) When Jake first stepped into leadership, the pressures of the job were intense—deadlines, decisions, a constant stream of responsibilities. He remembers one moment when he felt especially underwater. His leader, Brian, didn't offer quick fixes. Instead, he invited Jake into a conference room with a blank wall and a pack of yellow sticky notes. "Let's write it all out," Brian said. Each sticky note represented a responsibility or stressor. Brian helped make sense of the chaos. "What's most important here?" he asked. "What could be delegated? What's draining you that we could change?"

That personalized attunement offered Jake clarity, and years later, Jake found himself paying that moment forward. A team member came to him visibly frustrated, saying that he felt like he was doing more than he was hired to do. Jake didn't rush to justify or defend the workload. Instead, he pulled out the team member's job description and walked him to a whiteboard. "Let's take a look," he said. They spent the next hour mapping out tasks and sorting through expectations. Does this align with your role? Is there something here that someone else should own? By the end of the session, the team member felt lighter. Heard. Valued. This approach, Jake now believes, is what makes the difference between frustration and forward momentum. Or, as Bob Chapman, CEO of Barry-Wehmiller, puts it, "Management is about telling people what to do. Leadership is about caring for your people."

For many young people in Hughes's class, it's their first-ever experience of attunement in the workplace. But just that single experience can become a foundation for greater, more fulfilling success. Consider Kyanna, who started her career at Jersey Mike's at the age of sixteen and gradually advanced to become a franchise owner by the age of twenty-six. Or Austin, who started as a part-time employee in 2014, owned his first store by 2019 and eventually oversaw more than sixty locations across ten states. Once someone sees that they can be met with support, Hughes said, "They change. They listen to others more intently and coach their employees more intentionally. They lead differently."

Invest in them

We often treat personal development as something meant only for children, as though adulthood signals a completed and fully formed self. This belief is wrong and limiting. Renowned psychologist Erik Erikson argued that growth continues across our lifespans, and he identified midlife as a critical phase of "generativity"—a stage defined by our drive to contribute, mentor, and invest in the success of others, especially the next generation. When this drive is stifled, he warned, we risk slipping into "stagnation." In the workplace, stagnation can creep in slowly through missed promotions, a lack of learning opportunities, or roles that never evolve no matter how much we do. Over time, these small moments of neglect add up, fueling disengagement, resentment, and a lack of motivation. It's no surprise, then, that a 2021 Pew Research study found that one in three employees who left their jobs cited the absence of advancement opportunities as a key reason for quitting.

On the other hand, when employees are given chances to learn, stretch, and grow, they're far more engaged, more satisfied in their lives, and less likely to feel stuck. Investing in employees through mentorship, training, or clear pathways bolsters healthy adult development and sends a powerful message to them that they and their future matter here. Research finds that employees who feel they're growing are twice as likely to say they plan to stay with their organization for the long haul.

Mattering leaders understand this. Out of all the interviews I conducted for this book, perhaps the most striking example of a leader who invests in the development of people was Chuck Drury, the CEO of Drury Hotels. When it was time to create company-wide operating procedures, Chuck involved housekeepers, maintenance techs, and frontline managers—those who know the work best. By giving people who might not usually get this opportunity the chance to contribute, Chuck was investing in their growth and turning their experience and insights into the backbone of the company's policies. One key initiative is the President's Council, which brings frontline workers directly into leadership conversations, giving them space to grow professionally and shape the company's future. This investment is clearly working, evidenced by their employee retention. To date, the only people Chuck has ever lost from his senior management team are those who retired.

The company also invests in its employees by providing emergency financial support when they need it. In 2016, they created a hardship assistance program called INNTouch, which supports team members facing unexpected financial hardships, such as medical bills or a death in the family. The program has supported over 1,200 team members, signaling to Drury employees that they are worth real investment.

Emphasis on employee investment permeates not only across leadership but across the entire company. Take Saralee, a Drury employee and President's Council member I met with, who has a remarkable and inspiring story. When Saralee first interviewed for a housekeeping position at Drury, she had just left an abusive relationship and was struggling to make ends meet. "I had a lot of strikes against me," she recalled. "I was sixty-six, living in a crisis center. I had no experience in hotels. I'm relying on public transportation. Who's going to want me? Probably nobody." But her interviewer, Manuel, didn't react like she feared he would. Instead, he saw in Saralee someone with a good work ethic, someone worth investing in. The work had a definite learning curve, but Saralee's managers were patient with her, and soon she was excelling in the role, just as Manuel had predicted.

After a year of working as a housekeeper, Saralee was tapped to become a supervisor. To Saralee, each new role was an opportunity to learn, grow, and prove the value of Drury's ongoing investment. As a supervisor, Saralee is intentional about managing her team with the same generosity of investment Drury has shown her. "I've had to learn to give people grace, to be creative about bringing out the best in them, even when they're struggling," she said. Reflecting on her journey, she added, "Drury didn't just give me a job—they gave me a chance to grow. Because they believed in me, I started believing in myself—and now I'm helping others do the same."

> *Work, among all its abstracts, is actually intimacy, the place where the self meets the world. . . . Work is the inside made into the outside.*
>
> —David Whyte

Investing in people requires us to let go of the "taker" mindset that so often characterizes anti-mattering workplaces. As Wharton management professor Adam Grant explains, "Takers are people who, when they walk into an interaction with another person, are trying to get as much as possible from that person and contribute as little as they can in return, thinking that's the shortest and most direct path to achieving their own goals."

Grant's research reveals that "givers," on the other hand, seek opportunities to assist others, whether it's through introductions, advice, mentoring, or knowledge sharing, without any strings attached.

One executive who helped me understand how to shift from a taker to a giver mindset at work was Pietro Mangione, who left his home country of Italy to step into a leadership role at the consulting company Accenture in Australia. The pace was relentless. Days were filled with back-to-back meetings and urgent deadlines, and the international transition was proving overwhelming for him and his family. He soon became, by his own admission, a taker, keeping his head down, protecting himself, believing that if he didn't look out for his interests, no one else would. Outwardly, he projected confidence. But inside, he was burning out and probably even depressed, he said. His mindset made him feel isolated, constantly defensive, and focused on self-preservation rather than forming connections.

Pietro decided to quit. But before he could hand in his notice, something unexpected happened. He opened up that he was struggling, and a handful of senior leaders and friends offered support and mentorship. They talked about their own challenges in adapting to a new country. Their encouragement and belief in his potential convinced Pietro to stay. What they modeled, being so open and honest, changed how Pietro approached his own leadership. He wanted to invest in his colleagues the same way they had invested in him.

Pietro began small by carving out time in every team meeting for each person to share something real from their life, such as a recent win, a challenge they were working through, or something they were grateful for. Pietro would then use the insights from these conversations to connect his colleagues with mentors or suggest stretch assignments and professional development beyond their current roles. He made sure that every person knew that their growth mattered to him and that he was willing to invest real time, resources, and belief in their development.

This investment paid off. His team grew more cohesive and more successful because they felt supported to stretch and develop. Years later, a senior manager who, like Pietro, had relocated, thanked him for building a culture where she felt genuinely supported. "You've been a blessing to me and probably the most impactful person in my career this year," she wrote. "I've learned so much from you, Pietro . . . how you prioritize people and relationships. . . . You have been an example as a colleague and a leader." Reading her message, Pietro was struck by how drastically he had transformed. The taker had become an investor.

It's often said that people don't leave companies—they leave bad managers. And the flip side is equally true—that people stay for leaders who see them, support them, and help them grow. Pietro came to see how investing in your people yields even greater rewards. By leading with mattering, he built better teams *and* grew into a better version of himself. "In the end, our legacy is built not just on our own success and achievements," Pietro told me, "but on the success and achievements of those we helped along the way."

The long arm of the job

Ultimately, the mattering workplace is a countercultural space. It represents a deliberate rejection of the forces that have turned too many modern workplaces into a relentless, depleting, and dehumanizing grind. The average person spends one-third of their life at work. Work shapes how we see ourselves, the impact we can make in the world, and even our health. Researchers call it "the long arm of the job." When we feel like we don't matter at work, whether we're overlooked, micromanaged, or excluded from meaningful decisions, it takes a toll on the body, including a higher risk of cardiovascular disease, anxiety, and even early death.

The effects follow us home, too. Something called "the spillover-crossover model" confirms what many of us already know, that when work leaves us depleted, it becomes harder to be present for the people we love. Stress spills over into our personal lives and crosses over into our relationships, shaping how we parent and how we treat those closest to us. When we don't feel like we matter during the day, we often return home physically present but emotionally unavailable. Psychologists call this "proximal separation"—the emotional distance that forms when a parent is physically near but emotionally elsewhere, too overwhelmed or distracted to truly be present with their child. Our children sense it. And over time, in the absence of attunement, they may begin to believe that the disconnection is their fault, that something must be wrong with them.

On the other hand, when someone feels trusted, supported,

and empowered at work, they carry that sense of stability and energy into their personal relationships. Their inner reserves aren't depleted just trying to survive the day. Instead, they have the capacity to nurture their personal relationships. They are better able to be the parents, partners, and friends they want to be.

In fact, the long arm of the job doesn't stop at home. Some scholars argue that when we feel heard and our needs at work are considered, we carry that sense of mattering into our communities. A person who feels they can shape outcomes in their work environment is more likely to believe they can do the same elsewhere. That belief becomes a catalyst for engagement and fosters a kind of civic confidence. The person who feels empowered at work is more likely to, say, organize a blood bank during a local crisis, rally neighbors around a shared cause, or speak up at a city council meeting. Simply put, when people feel like they matter at work, they're more likely to believe they matter to the world around them.

CHAPTER 8

Be an Architect: Mattering Spaces

My black cab pulled up to the Bedford, a corner pub in a neighborhood in South London, and let me out on a sidewalk filled with strollers, young children on scooters, and neighbors pausing to chat. This pub, like so many in the UK, was like a magnet, pulling together the community around it. As I strolled along the sidewalk, I, too, felt the familiar pull I experience every time I visit London, a city that has become a second home to me.

Years earlier, as newlyweds, Peter and I moved to a neighborhood just a twenty-minute ride away. As excited as I was to be living in London, it was a lonely transition for me. I'd stepped away from a job I loved and close friends I'd known for decades to move with Peter to a new country with no work lined up (except for a little freelancing), no close friends, and no community. A few weeks in, I struggled with too many unstructured days—no place to be, no one depending on me, no one even looking for me.

Back then, I didn't yet understand how belonging to a place could buffer against loneliness. But I had hints of it. One evening, as I walked home with groceries hanging from my arm, I remember passing our local Chelsea pub, the Anglesea Arms, and finding myself lingering on the sidewalk to watch the patrons laughing and bonding inside. What I longed for on that winter evening was a familiar place like this pub, a space outside my house where I felt like I was a part of something bigger.

Now, years later, I was back in London, trying to answer the question that has stayed with me all these years, namely, Why do some public spaces make people feel a sense of belonging, while others remain strictly transactional? And what would it take to tip a public space into something that could build up our sense of mattering? A London-based researcher I interviewed suggested that I check out the Bedford and its unusually intentional approach to creating community.

As I stepped through the Bedford's heavy wooden doors, I walked past traditional pub tables and a well-worn, horseshoe-shaped bar. Becky, the head of events, greeted me with a bubbly hello. "Come with me quickly to the Club Room," she said, taking me by the arm. "It'll give you a sense of what we do here."

Without windows, the clubroom gave off a moody, middle-of-the-night vibe. It was five p.m., and there was a happy hour event going on, with loud music being played by a DJ and disco lights of colorful LED bulbs rotating patterns around the room. I was surprised to find that the dance floor was filled with *toddlers*—all of them rocking to the music, jamming with drums and tambourines. At the bar off to the side, strollers had taken the place of barstools. In about an hour's time, Becky told me, the toddler dance party would empty out, and the pub would set up for the Banana Cabaret comedy club, a show that would last until ten thirty p.m. After that, the room would clear again, this time to become a nightclub, until two a.m. The following day, the room would host a child's birthday party. Or, just as likely, it might be the site of a wake, a christening, or a wedding. For many of us, a pub evokes only images of drinking and casual socializing, but I was quickly realizing that there was something more nuanced and significant happening at the Bedford.

In talking to Becky, I learned that the COVID-19 pandemic had taken a toll on the pub. As news of the pandemic spread throughout the UK, Becky began to receive numerous cancellations. In just one day, £100,000 worth of events had been called off. Soon, she said, her once-loved job began to feel more like a nightmare. No longer feeling needed there, Becky resigned from the pub and took a job at a hospital specializing in mental health care, determined to support those who needed it most.

About six months later, Becky was walking her son to nursery school when she saw a ten-year-old girl crying on a bridge. Becky showed the girl her National Health Service lanyard and asked what was wrong. The girl explained she had run away from her foster parent and was trying to find her mom. Becky helped bring her to safety. The experience stayed with Becky. She decided to train as a child therapist. In October 2021, Becky started a postgraduate certificate in therapeutic play, helping children cope with issues ranging from bereavement to parents with alcohol addiction.

But, in the midst of her training, Becky had an epiphany. She could do more therapeutic work in hospitality—in a setting like a pub—than by serving a few private clients each week. The future of making mental health resources scalable, she believes, is by finding ways to support people in the context of their community. She calls what she does at the Bedford "pub therapy," integrating mental health support into daily life by creating a space where regulars can feel supported through life's inevitable ups and downs. She offers parents a welcoming place to gather with their children, provides elderly patrons a reason to leave home, and ensures that people who might otherwise feel isolated have a place where they feel like they belong.

Looking around the pub, I could see why Becky called it "pub therapy." Connections were happening all around me. A young couple was having an animated conversation at one table. Nearby, two older women shared a pot of tea and an occasional belly laugh. A man with his necktie loosened sat at the bar, chatting easily with the bartender as if they were old friends. In the corner, a group of gentlemen in their eighties rested their canes against the bar, alternating between conversation and comfortable silence. I learned from these men that they have been coming to the Bedford and sitting at those very stools for sixty years.

What felt powerful was how this seemingly ordinary public setting became a site of closeness and belonging for such a wide range of people. And by coming into this space, we were all, in one way or another, closer. Together, we were inhabiting time and sharing a close space, from shifting past each other at the bar to leaning in to be heard over the noise to passing pints and plates. We tend to think of mattering as an inner emotional experience. But maybe, I thought, what I was seeing and feeling at the Bedford pointed to something more, that there was a *physical* dimension to mattering, too. Was simply being in proximity to one another reinforcing mattering in ways we didn't recognize?

Find a third space

For years, sociologists have talked about the importance of third spaces as an antidote to the isolation of modern life. These are places outside our home (the first space) and work (the second space) where we can gather or simply just be in one another's presence. Third spaces include libraries, coffee shops, theaters, and gyms, the kind of low-profile places where we have informal interaction. These spaces matter for our sense of well-being. According to the Survey Center on American Life, people who engage in social interactions in third spaces report higher levels of happiness and life satisfaction.

More Spaces, More Friends: In 2024, the Survey Center on American Life found that there's a surprisingly close relationship between the density of civic spaces and friendship networks. "Americans with less access to civic infrastructure—such as parks, coffee shops, and libraries—have many fewer friends and

> report greater difficulty making social connections," noted the researchers. "Americans with no access to public or commercial places are more than three times more likely than those with the most access to report having no close friends (32 percent vs. 9 percent)."

And yet, our third spaces are dwindling, the casualty of expensive overhead, underinvestment, and events like the pandemic. We have more pop-ups and "experiences" but fewer reasons to be regulars somewhere. Increasingly, life online keeps us home. I thought about this as I stood in the pub and recalled how civic researcher Sam Pressler said it's not enough to just have third spaces. We also have to be intentional about how connection—or mattering, as I would put it—happens there. "We need to understand *where* people experience community, *how* people participate in it, and with *whom* they form relationships," he writes.

Pressler's civic infrastructure framework offers a way of analyzing the spaces around us. At first glance, the Bedford's eclectic mix of people and events might seem scattered. But the longer I was there, moving from activity to activity, the more I detected a sense of intention. The *where* of the Bedford was important: nestled in the heart of the neighborhood, a familiar place positioned where people naturally passed by on their way home from work or school. The *who* was just as considered: a multigenerational mix of neighbors that included retirees, young families, longtime locals, and newcomers. And then there was the *how*: The programming was the real secret sauce to the place, with Becky-curated events such as bridge club, a parents' morning meetup, game nights, and even choir practice.

After Becky showed me around, she took me to meet Ethan, the pub's general manager. Ethan had originally thought he would go into ministry, preaching on Sundays and shepherding a congregation. He'd gone to a Catholic seminary and become an ordained priest. But like Becky, he decided that the impact he wanted to have could happen in a more casual way. Eventually, he had found himself here. If Becky was doing "pub therapy," Ethan was doing what he called "pub ministry," connecting sincerely with everyone who walked in, remembering a regular's drink order, offering a listening ear, and noticing when someone was struggling. In our conversation, I could see how much it fulfilled him. "It's about serving and tending to people where they already are, making sure they know there's someone who cares about them, who is here to listen," Ethan said. He had translated his calling into something rooted in people's everyday lives.

> *Do your little bit of good where you are: it's those little bits of good put together that overwhelm the world.*
>
> —Desmond Tutu

Both Becky and Ethan thought strategically about the pub and the people in it. Much as architects think about functionality, flow, and design, they thought about their space with intention, not just as a business and not just as *any* space, but as a space where they could facilitate mattering. It made me think of the Danish architect Jan Gehl, who is famously responsible for transforming Copenhagen's busy streets into pedestrian-friendly third spaces filled with seating, bike lanes, shops, and sidewalks for people to interact. His approach in creating a space expressly for human connection was much like Becky and Ethan's. They weren't designing blueprints, but they were designing the connections within the pub.

In this way, we, too, can be architects of mattering. We may not run a pub or redesign a city, but we all move through physical spaces that we have the power to shape, from homes and offices to classrooms and coffee shops to parks and backyards. Thinking intentionally about space, as in how we create it, how we physically show up, and how we make others feel there, is a practice that can mediate mattering for ourselves and others in lasting ways. "We shape our buildings and afterwards our buildings shape us," said Sir Winston Churchill in a 1943 speech. He was speaking about the need to rebuild the bombed-out House of Commons, but his observation about our reciprocal relationship to buildings nevertheless captures something for us. We have the power to be architects, to design spaces for mattering, and those spaces, in turn, can shape our own mattering, too.

Define a space

You don't have to build a new space to think like a mattering architect. Instead, you can designate a space where you intentionally practice mattering by tuning in to others, opening yourself up to reliance, and engaging in mutual investment. Maybe it's your front stoop that holds a pair of chairs, making it easy to have an impromptu conversation with a neighbor. Maybe it's the park bench at the dog run, where a shared nod with someone you see every day turns into a conversation and eventually transforms into a trusted friendship. By being intentional about how you use these spaces, you can create the conditions for mattering to unfold. With time and consistency, these ordinary spots become mattering spaces because of the way people feel in them.

With time, your efforts may very well have a multiplicative effect. In San Francisco, Patty Smith and her husband declared the sidewalk in front of their building their "stoop," drinking their morning coffee in folding chairs every Saturday. Then a neighbor sat with them. After another few months, so many "stoopers" had joined them that the group threw a pancake party for the neighborhood. In Excelsior Springs, Missouri, Lisa and Mark Walter learned about a tradition known as "Flamingo Friday," a practice in which a host designates a gathering space by staking two pink plastic birds in a neighborhood yard. The Walters bought two flamingos of their own and invited friends and neighbors to come by their street on summer Fridays. Sometimes, just a handful of people appear. Other times, there are close to thirty. Wherever the flamingos are, people show up. In other words, by defining a third space—where everyone is equal, where people can be regulars, where interactions can reveal needs and build mutual investment—you can support mattering surprisingly effectively.

> The US is in a party deficit, notes writer Ellen Cushing. Only 4.1 percent of Americans attended or hosted a social event on an average weekend or holiday in 2023, according to the Bureau of Labor Statistics. Cushing writes, "Resolve to throw two parties—two because two feels manageable, and chain-letter math dictates that if every party has at least 10 guests (anything less is not a party!) and everyone observes host-guest reciprocity (anything else is sociopathic!), then everyone gets 20 party invitations a year—possibly many more. They do not need to be expensive, or formal, or in your own home. All you have to do is invite people in."

David Burton in Missouri used his driveway as a mattering space. Although he had lived in his neighborhood for eighteen years and had once been a regular participant in pickup basketball games, he noticed that as others moved away and life became busy with children, he actually knew only one neighbor. While he didn't throw loud parties and he was always sure to pick up after his dog, he realized that he had not been a particularly good neighbor. He and his wife decided to change that. They agreed to make an effort to be more neighborly by introducing themselves to their eight most immediate neighbors by ringing doorbells and delivering each a plate of homemade cookies. "We know you've lived here five years, and we've never spoken to you," they said to one. "But we want to do better." After that, they made an effort to greet people by name and engage them in small talk. These small gestures created a reciprocal spark. Others began greeting and involving themselves in neighborhood conversations, too. "I didn't know my neighbors, but it turned out my neighbors didn't know their neighbors," said David. As their exchanges became more frequent, David began inviting people to bring lawn chairs over for a driveway chat. There was no fancy hosting, David said. The purpose was simply to create a designated space where people could get talking.

When David's wife was diagnosed with cancer, neighbors rallied around her with practical help and encouragement. Many of them had their own experience with the disease and knew how to communicate empathy and importance. People now ask the couple to watch their dog or get the paper when they're out of town. David has started a Rotary club as another way of bringing people together. At the University of Missouri, where he works, he has even developed an extension course called "Neighboring 101" to teach others how to get to know their immediate eight neighbors—and others.

When Alex Hoskyn had her first baby, Henry, new parenthood left her feeling isolated. As a social worker who was used to having many conversations a day, she missed connecting with adults. To get out of the house, Alex took her baby to cafés around her town of Oldham, in England, but few people interacted with them. It surprised her that even being out of the house, you could still feel so lonely.

One day, Alex was sitting with Henry when she noticed a man

with a disability and his caregiver at a nearby table, looking like they'd run out of conversation. At another table, an elderly lady sat alone. Alex later thought, *Maybe if we had all sat together, we might have cheered each other up a bit.* She wasn't searching for lifelong friends, just company and conversation. She guessed that simply twenty minutes of informal connection would have made everyone happier.

In April 2017, Alex approached café owners with a proposal. Would they be open to designating a table for customers who want to chat over tea? Alex gave them a sign to put on the table, brochures explaining the idea of the "Chatty Cafe Scheme," and posters to put up. The idea took off. As café owners designated "chatty tables," people began to sit at them. Some cafés had to grow the size of their chatty tables to accommodate more people.

Before long, the concept spread across the UK to more than two thousand chatty cafés. It has also caught on in Poland, Gibraltar, Australia, Canada, and the US. Alex often hears from volunteers who take ownership of maintaining the tables in their corner of the world. Setting up a table is "one of the best things I did in 2023," one wrote. In a TEDx Talk, Alex told the story of Joan and Sarah, who started talking at a chatty café. "Within twenty minutes, thirty-year-old Sarah could tell you more about sixty-five-year-old Joan than she could about any of her work colleagues."

Alex's chatty cafés reminded me of Grandma Peggy and her breakfast guests. Grandma Peggy and the high schoolers experienced a weekly boost mediated not just by attunement but also by being in a specific space, her dining room table. The two gen-

erations might otherwise not have had much of a reason to interact. But over a table full of bacon, they developed a lasting bond.

Commit to a space

You might be wondering, What if I don't have the capacity to
create a space right now? What if I'm not particularly chatty or
don't want to buy flamingos? The beauty of being a mattering
architect is that it does not require that you generate the blueprint. You can invest in a space you already go to, like a yoga class
or the Saturday morning farmers' market.

For a few years, my dad went to the same casual restaurant
once a week for lunch. He learned the staff's names and took an
interest in their lives. When his mother-in-law—my nana—fell
ill, he stopped going for a while to help my mother care for her.
After my nana passed away, he returned to this restaurant, and
the staff greeted him with a sympathy card. He was so touched
that they had made the effort to go to a stationery store to buy a
card and by the thoughtfulness each of them showed in their personal note of condolence. By expressing care for the employees
of that restaurant, my dad had made such a strong impression in
that space that they felt his absence. The card underscored how
much he mattered there.

Showing up to the same pub or restaurant every week may
not feel like a particularly transformative act, but the regularity
of the practice does encode something in our bodies. Our brains
enjoy familiarity, a phenomenon that researchers have termed
"the mere exposure effect." It's the idea that repeated experiences

with sights, scents, sounds, and faces can make us feel safe. Even more, there's something uniquely grounding about the warmth of a hand, the power of eye contact, and the sound of a familiar voice. These actions trigger the release of oxytocin, the hormone that helps us feel connected and relaxed.

> An MIT study of college dorm friendships found that a big predictor of who became close friends wasn't shared interests but the distance between rooms. Students who lived closest to each other were far more likely to become close, while each additional doorway between them reduced their chances of forming a bond.

Standing in the pub—smelling the beer, hearing footsteps across the wood floor—I was struck by how mattering, too, relies on our nervous system. That desire for physical interaction is partly why modern life can feel so lonely. Fewer people gather in shared spaces like churches. Much of our shopping has moved online. Even our social time gets compressed into quick texts. But being physically present naturally increases our awareness of each other. It helps us connect to our impact by revealing, through others' tone of voice and body language, the effect our actions have on others. Even our own physical needs, like needing comfort, can help cue us for reliance, and whether those needs are met often defines how we feel prioritized or not. Some of the benefits of in-person connection just can't be replaced by screens.

Throw up scaffolding

To create a mattering space, sometimes you need scaffolding, the lightweight, flexible assistance that helps you and others "grow into" this space. In other words, you need materials that help people linger, open up, maybe go deeper, and, most of all, want to return. For this, do not underestimate the power of food. The experience of eating or drinking together is powerfully binding. It reduces social pressure, creates a shared sensory experience, and, if all else fails, gives us an out if we need it. ("I'm heading to the bar to get another drink.") It's also an incredible motivator. Announce that there will be cookies at the next meeting, and you'll almost always have more people come and stay. The presence of food, research finds, acts as a "social glue." It signals generosity, abundance, informality, and intimacy, all elements that prime us for connection.

> **Table Talk:** In French, *copain* (friend) and in Italian *compagno* (companion) come from the Latin *cum pānis*, literally "with-bread." The Chinese term for partner, 伙伴, stems from a similar term (火伴), which translates to "fire mate," a reference to sharing meals over a campfire.

You do not need to be a master chef or put out a giant spread for food to serve as scaffolding. Maybe you keep extra sparkling waters in your fridge and cookies in the freezer that you can re-heat at a moment's notice. Or maybe you share soup, as Hope Murphy did in Maine. One year, as winter rolled in, she thought about how she loved making soup but got tired of the leftovers. Wouldn't it be cool if we could swap leftovers? she thought. So, she invited friends to each cook a pot of their favorite soup to share on the second Sunday of every month. Her friends didn't all know each other, but after the first gathering, this twist on the potluck became a winter tradition. Soon, they all took turns hosting. "What I love most about these soup suppers is that we all own this event," Hope said to a local reporter. "It's not me entertaining, or whoever is hosting it; the soup suppers belong to all of us."

At the Bedford pub, where food and drink are already plenti-ful, Becky introduced a board game night because she recognized that joint play can be just as powerful a binding agent as food. Play, studies find, breaks down barriers, creates enjoyment with-out the pressure of small talk, and gives people a low-stakes way to invest in others. Games like Catan and Ticket to Ride brought in a new crowd, eventually growing into thirty regulars. Becky's instincts around the connective power of in-person play are echoed in the rise of board game cafés, where chains like Snakes & Lattes and any number of individual spots—like the Rook & Pawn, in Athens, Georgia, or Empire Board Game Library, in Al-buquerque, New Mexico—have been purposely designed as spaces where people can eat *and* play. The steady rise of these cafés seems to be tapping into a growing desire for real, face-to-face connection.

Think creatively about your scaffolding. It might even center around an idea. Not long ago, a group of women invited me to join what you might think of as an article club, like a book club but with a lighter lift. The structure is simple. Once a month, one of us hosts lunch in our kitchen. Each gathering has clear scaffolding. We share a meal, and we come prepared to discuss the same news article that we selected ahead of time. Some people cook from scratch; others (like me) order in. While the article gives us a focal point, a reason to gather, the real magic happens in what unfolds around it. Our conversations inevitably spill into stories about our families, the messiness of middle age, the demands of work, and the state of the world. What's extraordinary about this group is that many of us didn't know each other before it was created. It's a group made of friends of friends, and yet, by being intentional, we were able to build the kind of trust that, at least I once thought, would take years to develop. As one woman in our group so beautifully put it, we made a choice to embrace new people and built a little community. "It is not easy—it took time no one has; it was a risk in that regard because we all tangibly appreciate the price of time," she said. "But we did it, and it found its place. It met a need I didn't know I had." By prioritizing these once-a-month meetups and each other, we nurture and protect this mattering space. If one of us has to miss a meeting, we all feel her absence.

Not from scratch

To create a mattering space, sometimes we just need to get more intentional about how we use the spaces we already have. When twenty-seven-year-old Kelli Johnson studied abroad in Europe, she saw laundromats acting as communal spaces. Many of them had adjoining cafés. She knew she wanted to bring the concept back home to Milwaukee, Wisconsin. After graduating with a degree in natural resources and environmental studies, she pursued the idea. She got many noes from laundromat owners not looking to sell but finally got her yes from the owner of a little laundromat in a quiet neighborhood. The space was dusty, with aging machines, but Johnson had a vision to make it into a third space.

Little by little, she gave the Washroom a new life, painting green checkers on the floors, adding colorful backsplash to the walls, and creating a little library for people to take and leave books. She also stocked a vending machine with snacks and atypical items like tarot cards, stickers, condoms, and Narcan. "This is an area with a lot of college students who might need those things for cheap," she said, "so I'm making sure they feel welcome." She hosts a free wash-and-dry day—"No questions asked, you come in and wash your clothes"—and has invited local artists to decorate the Washroom's walls.

Mattering Nudges: In response to growing loneliness among elderly customers, the Dutch supermarket chain Jumbo introduced slow checkout lanes, where cashiers in this lane are encouraged to take extra time to chat, especially with older customers. This simple buffer against loneliness has now spread to about two hundred stores. It's with small, intentional changes like this that we can begin to scale mattering and embed it into everyday lives.

Kelly has noticed people sticking around and interacting with one another. A student named Tony comes to the Washroom simply for a place to think. "I never thought that I'd be saying, like, 'Oh, I'm gonna go to the laundromat just to be there,'" he said. Another customer, Rachel, always brings a book to read while she hangs out. One evening, she noticed that a couple doing their laundry brought their cat, which they kept outside on a harness. Rachel had been trying to figure out how to leash-train her kitten and took this as an opportunity to chat, leaving with some helpful tips.

Kelly has ideas to transform the Washroom into a more communal space, but for now, she finds joy in the friendly texts she frequently receives from customers expressing their enjoyment. One person told her they'd chosen the Washroom for their first date. On the security camera, she's also noticed a regular who likes to dance to the music she plays. "He comes in with just the best vibe ever," she said.

Scale mattering

When we actively invest in third spaces, we can turn them into mattering engines, rippling outward and strengthening the social fabric of entire communities. That was Lorenzo Lewis's vision when he set out to use barbershops as a way to support the mental health of Black men in his hometown of Little Rock, Arkansas. Born to an incarcerated mother and raised by relatives, Lorenzo knew what it felt like to struggle without emotional support. When he discovered Barbershop Books, an initiative that placed children's libraries in barbershops, it sparked an idea. Lorenzo wondered whether barbershops could become places to address emotional health, too. What if, Lorenzo thought, these comfortable and familiar spaces, where Black men already gathered to talk about sports, family, and life, could also be places for open conversations about mental health? What if barbers, already trusted members of their communities, were trained to identify signs of emotional distress in their clients? If they were equipped to guide conversations about mental health, to listen deeply, and to validate experiences, they could play a meaningful role in breaking the stigma that kept so many Black men from seeking help in the first place.

When Lorenzo met Matt Dillon at Goodfellas Barbershop in Little Rock, Matt immediately saw his vision and agreed to let Lorenzo try to lead a conversation about mental health among the clients in his barbershop. A few days later, Lorenzo sat in Matt's shop surrounded by the sounds of clippers buzzing and scissors snipping and waited for a natural pause in the conversation. When the moment came, Lorenzo took a deep breath and jumped in. "Guys, I just want to have a conversation about life."

The room grew quieter as he shared his story. He explained being born to an incarcerated mother and growing up with parents who struggled with addiction. "I know I'm not the only one who's been through something like this," he said. A few of the men began to nod knowingly. Then, one by one, they started to share their own stories—struggles with absent fathers, brushes with the law, and the need to stay strong in the face of constant challenges. Lorenzo's "confession" had created a space where others felt safe to express their own "confessions," too. The barber's chair, once a place for casual conversation, had become something deeper, a place where men could feel seen and understood. In that conversation, the Confess Project was born.

Drawing on therapy-informed approaches, Lorenzo and his team have developed a research-validated training program that equips barbers with four core techniques to better support their clients' emotional well-being. First, they're taught empathetic listening, which involves tuning in to subtle changes in a client's mood or behavior and responding with care. Second, they're instructed how to engage in positive communication, using affirming words that recognize a client's strength and resilience. Third, they're trained to pick up nonverbal communication, using eye contact, a calm tone, and presence to show genuine care. Fourth, they're shown how to guide clients to mental health resources when they are in crisis. Lorenzo told me the story of a man who confided to his barber that he didn't want to live. Because of his training, the barber stayed calm, listened, and then gently asked if he could call someone who could help. The man agreed, and a therapist responded within minutes. Lorenzo said that the act of tuning in and responding with care may have saved a life.

Today, the Confess Project has trained over four thousand barbers and beauty professionals in sixty-one cities and thirty-two states, reaching over 4 million people per year. After attending one of Lorenzo's training sessions in Delaware, I was convinced that you don't need to be a therapist to make a positive difference in someone's mental health. You just need a willingness to tune in, show you care, and start the conversation in a space that invites that kind of vulnerability.

Become a steward

Becoming a mattering architect expands your lens. Like Lorenzo, you might start considering how specific spaces can support mattering in your community and look for ways you can play a part. In 2017, when Shamichael Hallman was overseeing a multimillion-dollar renovation of Cossitt Library in downtown Memphis, he knew that to make the aging library a space for mattering, he needed to think beyond a shiny facelift. So he went to the neighbors to find out more about their genuine needs. "What do you need this library to be?" and "How could it help your daily life?" he asked.

The answers came quickly: a café for the food-scarce area, a marked space for artists and entrepreneurs, and a library with movable shelves and meeting spots that could adapt to the community's changing needs. Hallman helped with a redesign that also acknowledged the library's history as a former space of segregation, commissioning art and exhibits that told the story of the Memphis activists who had fought for desegregation. He also created new staff positions that didn't require library science degrees so that community members could work there. What was historically a building limited to the few has become a space for the many. Shamichael invites library-goers to enjoy themselves and to give back with their time or skills. "Stewardship of the space is important," he has said. "It has something to offer you, but you also have something to offer the space."

With the Bedford, Becky and Ethan have created a nerve center for a community and a living example of a mattering space. Take Alex, for example, a patron who rents the clubroom and main bar so that she can host workshops for new parents on weaning, baby first aid, and nutrition. It is difficult to find venues with enough space for all the baby strollers, she noted, and the pub—easy to get to, with coffee available—has that room. The pub has become an oasis for local parents, who aren't made to feel like an unhappy baby or frazzled caregivers are barriers to entry. One recent event, a talk and brunch with a psychotherapist, attracted thirty-eight new moms.

There's Nell, who teaches yoga at the pub on Mondays and Fridays. Many attendees are over the age of fifty. "I have a sweet man who comes to yoga, whose wife has early dementia. I used to teach her, and then when she couldn't come anymore, he came," she said. "It really is a community, and they're really dear souls."

When Nell split from her husband and was experiencing a difficult time, her students in turn supported her: "I can't describe how nurtured I felt by them."

And then there is Kit, who runs the bridge club. His work as an actor began dwindling as he aged. "When you're not getting auditions," he told me, "it can really bottom you out emotionally unless you have areas of your life where you feel like you matter." While he waited for callbacks, he decided to use his acting skills—active listening, a memory for information, and confidence—to bring people from the neighborhood together for bridge. "It's interesting, of course, that it's called bridge," he said, "because that's what it feels like: building new partnerships."

The Bedford bridge club list now has two hundred players. For many, the club is a place to make friendships that spill over into other areas of life. Some older widows, for example, met at the bridge table and started playing games at one another's houses, too. "I've also seen it be a lifeline for others who don't go out very much," he said.

In his youth, bridge clubs had established locations, but many have since shut down, and there are fewer and fewer community centers to host them, Kit said. "In the old days, the idea of running a bridge club in a pub would have been anathema," he told me. But the Bedford has everything: space, big rooms, tables and chairs, tea and coffee. "I wouldn't have thought there was such a need for this," he said, "but being in the middle of it, it now seems quite obvious that there is."

The Power of "We Matter"

As I was finishing this book, something happened that took the ground right out from under me. My kind, gentle father unexpectedly passed away. It started with a call from my sister, Natalie, to tell me that Dad had been rushed to the hospital with a complication from the Parkinson's disease he had been managing for the past few years. Less than twenty-four hours later, he passed away peacefully with my mom, my sister, and me by his side.

My father's death shook me to my core, and I mean this literally. In the days and weeks that followed, I felt myself shaking, like how you feel when you step outside on a cold day and the wind cuts through you. There was the immediate grief, the aching loss of him and how he made me feel safe and steady in the world. But underneath was a harder-to-name disorientation. It was the loss of someone who, along with my mom, had been the foundation of my mattering.

My parents made me feel seen from the very start. Whether

my dad and I were playing catch on our lawn, as we did every day after dinner when I was growing up, or my mother was tucking me in at night, my parents were a consistent and steady presence. A few years ago, while my dad and I were watching my kids play in the yard, I asked if he ever wished he could go back in time and relive our childhoods. He smiled and said gently, "When you're fully present, you don't really feel a need to go back." Being paid that kind of loving attention lodges deep inside your sense of self. It grounds you. When he died, it felt like part of my anchor went with him.

Loss touches all of us. Sometimes it occurs abruptly, and other times it unfolds gradually over time. Change, even when it is a good change, represents loss of what was, of who we were, of what we thought life would be. Sometimes society itself seems to shake us to our core. Maybe you are worried about making rent or the state of our planet. For many of us today, there's a constant sense of instability hovering just beneath the surface. It's easy to feel like the anchors we once counted on aren't there anymore, leaving us adrift.

In the days after my dad's passing, people from every chapter of his life began reaching out—texting, emailing, leaving notes on his online obituary—sharing story after story about the profound ways he impacted them. He had a rare gift for making people feel seen and valued, whether you were his grandchild or the person wrapping his order at the deli. He was incredibly humble in the way he moved through the world. He never once raised his voice—to anyone, ever. *How did he do that?* Can you imagine what the world would be like if everyone lived this way?

As I read these messages, it suddenly became clear. My dad had lived the mattering principles. He made people feel valued. A neighbor recalled my dad's countless small kindnesses over the years. He invested in people. My friends from high school wrote to me, remembering the advice and encouragement he'd offered them. He listened to people. One family friend wrote, "Pat was always attuned to the people around him, always making others know he wanted to hear their stories." My dad built a network of mattering that reverberated even after he was gone.

All of us have the power to do this. As we move through our days, we are shaping the lives around us, often without even realizing it. Each small kindness, each time we tune in and make someone feel seen and valued, we are building a mattering network. Over time, that network becomes stronger than any one individual. It holds and survives when change upends everything. It is this network of relationships that is the ultimate secret to sustaining our sense of mattering. Mattering isn't something we achieve on our own, stockpiled and tucked away somewhere to pull out when tough times come. It is something we create between us. It lives in our relationships, communities, and collective memory. And because of this, it doesn't disappear when we're no longer here. It lasts. By building up each other's sense of mattering, we secure our own. The outpouring of memories after my father's death was proof of that.

No one is finally dead until the ripples they cause
in the world die away, until the clock wound up
winds down, until the wine she made has finished

its ferment, until the crop they planted is harvested. The span of someone's life is only the core of their actual existence.

—Terry Pratchett

No matter what kind of upheaval we're facing, be it job loss, retirement, empty nesting, a shifting world, or some other destabilizing event, the surest way to sustain our own sense of mattering is to focus on making others feel like they matter. The shift from "I matter" to "we matter" gives us both the long-term resilience and legacy we crave. Over time, these small moments weave into something larger—a web of mattering that can catch us when the next wave of change hits.

As I struggled in the weeks after my dad's death, what held me together was the network I didn't fully realize I had until I needed it. Fueled by the care and support of others, I recommitted myself to passing on the gift my dad gave me. I returned to this book, more determined than ever, knowing that helping others feel valued is not small, or even big, work. It is *the* work. And that work can start with a gesture as simple as a clementine.

Now, every time I see clementines piled high in a market or tucked into a bowl on a kitchen table, I smile, thinking back to the shopkeeper at the Harlem train station. I remember the warmth of his bodega and the sense of mattering he offers his customers. Clementines serve as a reminder that one small, everyday act of care is how mattering takes root and grows into a movement.

———

Mattering has made my life richer in countless ways. It's made me want to be more intentional with the people I love, more present with my children, more thoughtful with my colleagues, and kinder to strangers I meet or pass on the street. I try to pay closer attention, ask better questions, and work hard to ensure no one around me feels like an afterthought. And when my own mattering takes a hit—when I feel overlooked, rejected, or unsteady—I now have the language to name it, the tools to cope, and a map to find my way back. My hope and belief is that it can do the same for you and those you care about.

Once you know what mattering can do, you'll start seeing it everywhere. And like my dad, you may find yourself wanting to help others feel it too. Too often, we hold back. We feel the nudge to reach out and say the thing that might lift someone up, but we hesitate, waiting for them to go first. The irony is, of course, that they're often waiting on us, too. In these moments, it is up to us to break through the inertia, to be willing to make that first move.

What I've learned through the hundreds of conversations I've had over these past six years is that, deep down, under all the loneliness, anxiety, and polarization—under all the things pulling us apart—we are all searching for the same thing.

We want to know that *who we are* and *what we do* make a difference in this world.

We want to know that our lives—our very existence—matters.

Acknowledgments

This book wouldn't exist without the tremendous support and investment of the many "cornermen" in my life.

To my wonderful agents, Christy Fletcher and Gráinne Fox—thank you for believing in the power of mattering from the very beginning. To my brilliant team at Portfolio—my publisher, Adrian Zackheim, and my editor extraordinaire, Niki Papadopoulos, whose vision, wisdom, and care are a gift to every author lucky enough to work with them. To my UK agent, Richard Pike, and editor at UK HarperCollins, Arabella Pike—thank you for your insights and support in bringing this book to readers in the UK.

Many thanks to my publicist Angela Baggetta, Original Strategies team, and the team at Portfolio—Margot Stamas, Jacqueline Galindo, Lucile Culver, Bonnie Sodek, Lauren Ball, Brian Lemus, Leila Sandlin, Amanda Lang, and everyone across marketing, publicity, design, and production. Your thoughtfulness and craftsmanship strengthened this book at every step. I am deeply grateful to Laura Crossley, who designed the iconic cover for this book.

It so perfectly captures the beauty, simplicity, and warmth of mattering.

This book benefited greatly from the extraordinary Verto team: Gareth Cook, Kate Rodemann, Chaz Curet, Eli Mannerick, and Elizabeth Winkler. Your collective genius, big hearts, and masterful edits helped shape every chapter. I couldn't have written this book without you. Thank you, too, to my remarkable researchers, Rachel Ryan, Tess Boosin, and Henry Rodin; my meticulous fact-checker, Laurie Flynn; and Michaela Corning-Myers for her diligent citation support.

I owe an enormous debt of thanks to the researchers of mattering, whose work is the basis of this book: Gregory Elliott, Gordon Flett, Julie Haizlip, Isaac Prilleltensky, Morris Rosenberg, and Nancy Schlossberg. Thank you for sharing your insights so generously. Thank you to Paul Rosenberg, who trusted me with his father Morris's unpublished chapters on mattering. I'd also like to thank researcher Marianne Etherson at the University of Glasgow in the UK for helping me draft my mattering survey questions and Michael Grugan at Northumbria University, Newcastle, for helping me interpret the data.

To my fellow cofounders of the Mattering Movement—Sarah Bennison, Kimberly Kravis, Kimberly Towner, and our illustrious advisory board and partners—thank you for seeing the potential of what mattering could offer the world and for bringing your expertise to amplify our important nonprofit work. To Tom Dunne and Meghan Lockwood at Harvard College, Rick Weissbourd at Harvard's Graduate School of Education, Lindsey Burghardt at Harvard's Center on the Developing Child, Rob Ernst and Lindsey

Acknowledgments

Mortenson at the University of Michigan, and Eleanor Daugherty and the team at Georgetown—I'm grateful for your partnership in helping young people know they matter.

To my friends who read early drafts of this book and offered meaningful and constructive feedback: Lisa Brancaccio, Courtney della Cava, Vicki Foley, Lisa Heffernan, Natalie and Pete Jones, Chris Pavone, Meredith Rollins, and Catherine Wallace. To friends who have engaged in long conversations about mattering for years: Michelle Aielli, Vanessa Bennett, Kelly Corrigan, Lisa Damour, Lizzie Weinreb Fishman, Ina Garten, Tira Grey, Dana and Michael Jones, Jenny and Matt Kabaker, Tara Kinsey, Beth Kojima, Cara Natterson, Aliza Pressman, Pilar Queen, Rebecca Raphael, and Rachel and John Rodin. To the wonderful Alexandra Leon, whose wisdom, creativity, and hard work keep our family organized. To the rest of my beloved village, I thank my lucky stars that I get to go through life with you. And to Katie Spikes, whose absence is felt daily and whose life was the embodiment of mattering.

To Lauren Lavelle—your brilliance and insights have added so much to this book, to my work, and to my life. How grateful I am to get to work side by side with you every day.

To my late father, Patrick, and my mother, Carole, thank you for giving me such a strong foundation in mattering and for passing that gift on to your six grandchildren with such love and intention. To my first and best friend, my sister Natalie, and my wonderful brother-in-law, Pete, thank you for the countless ways you support our family. I won the jackpot with you two, and I know it.

Acknowledgments

To my children, William, Caroline, and James, thank you for encouraging me to focus when I needed to write and for surrounding me with so much love throughout every stage of this journey. Your support made the hard process of writing a book much more meaningful and achievable. You matter to me more than any words can say.

To my husband, Peter, thank you for your endless encouragement and support, for taking on long stretches of being the lead parent, and for letting me borrow your courage whenever I need it. You bring so much fun, joy, and adventure to my life. What a privilege to get to be your partner.

To the hundreds of people who opened their hearts to me and trusted me to tell their stories, I am so grateful for your generosity. Your insights will change lives. They've already changed mine. It has been said that with the right words, you can change the world. Without a doubt, mattering can do just that.

Appendix: Mattering Assessment

The following self-assessment, based on research and insights from various surveys on mattering, is meant to get you thinking about your sense of mattering in the different domains of your life. As you read through each statement, notice your response. In which areas does your sense of mattering feel strong and secure, and which areas could use more nurturing? You can also use this reflection exercise to better understand someone you care about. Remember, mattering is something we can support, in ourselves and in others, through intentional actions.

Mattering to Myself

- **Recognition:** I acknowledge and value the positive impact I make on the world.

- **Reliance:** I know I can count on myself to follow through when it matters.

- **Importance:** I know how to prioritize my needs, even when life is busy.

- **Ego Extension:** I believe I am worthy of others' investment.

- **Attunement:** I understand my inner world and respond to myself with compassion.

Mattering to Friends and Family

- **Recognition:** My presence and contributions are noticed and valued by the people close to me.

- **Reliance:** People depend on me.

- **Importance:** Others make time for me and prioritize our relationship.

- **Ego Extension:** My loved ones are genuinely invested in my happiness and success, just as I am in theirs.

- **Attunement:** I feel understood and responded to by those closest to me.

Mattering at Work

- **Recognition:** My efforts at work are seen and acknowledged.

- **Reliance:** I have responsibilities that others depend on me to fulfill.

- **Importance:** My well-being is taken seriously.

- **Ego Extension:** I have someone at work who is invested in my growth.

- **Attunement:** I have someone at work who knows me well.

Mattering in Society

- **Recognition:** I believe my voice or actions make an impact in my community or society.

- **Reliance:** There are causes, groups, or people that rely on me and benefit from what I offer.

- **Importance:** I feel that I count and that I'm not just a bystander in the world.

- **Ego Extension:** I feel invested in the broader world and trust that, in its own way, the world is invested in me.

- **Attunement:** I feel that society understands, values, and responds to my needs with care, dignity, and respect.

If the ideas around mattering have resonated with you, please consider sharing them with others. This is how we can all become the "agents of mattering" our world so desperately needs right now.

Notes

Introduction: The Mattering Core

4 **value to add to the world:** Isaac Prilleltensky, "Mattering at the Intersection of Psychology, Philosophy, and Politics," *American Journal of Community Psychology* 65, no. 1–2 (2020): 16–34, pubmed.ncbi.nlm.nih.gov/31407358.

4 **Does my life make:** Community College of Rhode Island (CCRI), "Brown Professor Greg Elliott Speaks at CCRI's Professional Development Day Mattering," YouTube video, 54:48, from a talk presented by Greg Elliott on March 31, 2017, posted by CCRI, April 17, 2017, youtube.com/watch?v=1-iCaV6sy9w.

5 **mattering in the 1980s:** Morris Rosenberg and B. Claire McCullough, "Mattering: Inferred Significance and Mental Health Among Adolescents," *Research in Community & Mental Health* 2 (1981): 163–82, psycnet.apa.org/record/1983-07744-001.

5 **a single, intuitive concept:** Prilleltensky, "Mattering at the Intersection," 17.

5 **drives human behavior:** Rebecca Newberger Goldstein, "The Mattering Instinct: A Conversation with Rebecca Newberger Goldstein," *Edge*, March 16, 2016, edge.org/conversation/rebecca_newberger_goldstein-the-mattering-instinct.

6 *eudaimonia*, **the flourishing life:** Brian Duignan, "eudaimonia,"

Encyclopedia Britannica, last updated April 10, 2025, britannica
.com/topic/eudaimonia.

6 **foundational for well-being:** "Alfred Adler: Theory and
Application," Adler Graduate School, last updated 2021, alfredadler
.edu/about/alfred-adler-theory-application.

6 **The universal need:** Nancy K. Schlossberg, "Marginality and
Mattering: Key Issues in Building Community," *New Directions for
Student Services* 48 (1989): 4, https://doi.org/10.1002/ss.37119
894803.

8 **"Mattering is double-edged":** Gordon L. Flett, "An Introduction,
Review, and Conceptual Analysis of Mattering as an Essential
Construct and an Essential Way of Life," *Journal of Psychoeducational
Assessment* 40, no. 1 (2022): 3–36.

10 **A major driver of this trend:** Anne Case and Angus Deaton,
Deaths of Despair and the Future of Capitalism (Princeton
University Press, 2020).

10 **across 140 countries:** Ellyn Maese, "Almost a Quarter of the World
Feels Lonely," Gallup, October 24, 2023, news.gallup.com/opinion
/gallup/512618/almost-quarter-world-feels-lonely.aspx.

10 **Flett has termed "anti-mattering":** Gordon L. Flett et al., "The
Anti-Mattering Scale: Development, Psychometric Properties and
Associations with Well-Being and Distress Measures in Adolescents
and Emerging Adults," *Journal of Psychoeducational Assessment*
40, no. 1 (December 2021).

11 **"the essence of inhumanity":** George Bernard Shaw, *The Devil's
Disciple* (1896; Penguin Books, 1960).

11 **or thinking much about them:** Morris Rosenberg, unpublished
manuscript, undated, courtesy of Paul B. Rosenberg, MD.

Chapter 1: Connect to Your Impact

18 **"Do I matter to you?":** Oprah Winfrey, "Do I Matter?," YouTube
video, 01:28, from the Born This Way Foundation Launch Event,
posted by I CHOOSE PEOPLE, May 28, 2012, youtube.com/watch
?v=j33F8cVswqw.

19 **"the feeling that one":** Morris Rosenberg, unpublished manuscript, undated, courtesy of Paul B. Rosenberg, MD.

22 **"The deepest principle":** William James, *The Letters of William James*, vol. 2 (Boston: Atlantic Monthly Press, 1920), 33.

23 **the person behind an action:** Sara B. Algoe, Laura E. Kurtz, and Nicole M. Hilaire, "Putting the 'You' in 'Thank You': Examining Other-Praising Behavior as the Active Relational Ingredient in Expressed Gratitude," *Social Psychological and Personality Science* 7, no. 7 (June 2016).

27 **a survival tactic we inherited:** Catherine J. Norris, "The Negativity Bias, Revisited: Evidence from Neuroscience Measures and an Individual Differences Approach," *Social Neuroscience* 16, no. 1 (2021): 68–82.

29 **"put a man on the moon":** Andre M. Carton, "'I'm Not Mopping the Floors, I'm Putting a Man on the Moon': How NASA Leaders Enhanced the Meaningfulness of Work by Changing the Meaning of Work," *Administrative Science Quarterly* 63, no. 2 (2017): 323–69.

29 **"Do what you can":** Squire Bill Widener quoted in Theodore Roosevelt, *Theodore Roosevelt: An Autobiography* (Charles Scribner's Sons, 1920), 337.

29 **tend to cook better food:** Harvard Business Review Editors, "Cooks Make Tastier Food When They Can See Their Customers," *Harvard Business Review*, November 2014, hbr.org/2014/11/cooks-make-tastier-food-when-they-can-see-their-customers.

31 **ripple through our social networks:** James H. Fowler and Nicholas A. Christakis, *Connected: The Surprising Power of Our Social Networks and How They Shape Our Lives* (Little, Brown, 2009).

31 **Scottish poet Donna Ashworth:** Donna Ashworth, "YOU," excerpted from *Wild Hope* (Mango Publishing, 2023), donnaashworth.com/you.

Chapter 2: The Good Kind of Weight

39 **regular volunteering was linked:** David Mellor et al., "Volunteering and Well-Being: Do Self-Esteem, Optimism, and

Perceived Control Mediate the Relationship?," *Journal of Social Service Research* 34 (2008): 61–70.

40 **in control of our schedules:** Cassie Mogilner, "You'll Feel Less Rushed If You Give Time Away," *Harvard Business Review*, September 2012, hbr.org/2012/09/youll-feel-less-rushed-if-you-give-time-away.

40 **"The heavier the burden":** Milan Kundera, *The Unbearable Lightness of Being* (New York: Harper & Row, 1984).

43 **"The worst thing that could":** Kurt Vonnegut, *The Sirens of Titan* (Dial Press Trade Paperbacks, 1959).

46 **"the advice-giving effect":** Alison Wood Brooks and Francesca Gino, "Asking Advice Makes a Good Impression," *Scientific American*, October 7, 2014, scientificamerican.com/article/asking-advice-makes-a-good-impression.

46 **"richest sources of self-esteem":** Angela Chen, "A Social Psychologist Explains Why We Should Ask for Help More Often," *The Verge*, June 22, 2018, theverge.com/2018/6/22/17475134/heidi-grant-reinforcements-help-social-psychology.

49 **"The purpose of life":** Leo Rosten, speech at the National Book Awards, New York, 1962.

50 **Kohn's pangs of loneliness:** Noëlle de Leeuw, "Are You Lonely? Join These Women for a Walk in the Park," *Elle*, May 25, 2023, elle.com/life-love/a43990707/city-girls-who-walk-new-york-city.

55 **A small act can have:** Allison Rauch, "butterfly effect," *Encyclopedia Britannica*, last updated June 20, 2025, britannica.com/science/butterfly-effect.

Chapter 3: Mattering Too Much

62 **balance between adding value:** Isaac Prilleltensky, "Mattering at the Intersection of Psychology, Philosophy, and Politics," *American Journal of Community Psychology* 65, no. 1–2 (2020): 16–34, pubmed.ncbi.nlm.nih.gov/31407358.

63 **Gordon Flett calls importance:** Gordon Flett, "An Introduction, Review, and Conceptual Analysis of Mattering as an Essential

Construct and an Essential Way of Life," *Journal of Psychoeducational Assessment* 40, no. 1 (2021): 3–36, doi.org/10.1177/073428292 11057640.

66 **over the past fifty years:** "Raising Kids and Running a Household: How Working Parents Share the Load," Pew Research Center, November 4, 2015, pewresearch.org/social-trends/2015/11/04 /raising-kids-and-running-a-household-how-working-parents -share-the-load.

67 **Young people are feeling:** Richard Weissbourd et al., "Caring for the Caregivers: The Critical Link Between Parent and Teen Mental Health," Making Caring Common, June 2023, mcc.gse.harvard .edu/reports/caring-for-the-caregivers.

67 **overwhelming compared with other adults:** Office of the Surgeon General, *Parents Under Pressure: The U.S. Surgeon General's Advisory on the Mental Health & Well-Being of Parents*, US Department of Health and Human Services, 2024, ncbi.nlm.nih .gov/books/NBK606662.

69 **"our job is to be silent":** Amanda Sullender, "'Both Important and Secondary': Simone Gorrindo Examines Life as an Army Wife in New Memoir 'The Wives,'" *The Spokesman-Review*, April 14, 2024, spokesman.com/stories/2024/apr/14/both-important-and-secondary -simone-gorrindo-examp.

72 **"Self-care *is* other-focused":** Danna Thomas, *Happy Teacher Revolution: The Educator's Roadmap to Claiming and Sustaining Joy* (Jossey-Bass, 2024), 1.

73 ***Because it does:*** Becky Kennedy, "Mom Rage with Anna Mathur," *Good Inside with Dr. Becky*, July 26, 2022, goodinside.com/podcast /3789/mom-rage-with-anna-mathur.

74 **"I have always felt that":** James Baldwin and Richard Avedon, *Nothing Personal* (New York: Atheneum, 1964).

76 **reduced levels of cortisol:** Suniya S. Luthar et al., "Fostering Resilience Among Mothers Under Stress: 'Authentic Connections Groups' for Medical Professionals," *Women's Health Issues* 27, no. 3 (2017): 382–90.

77 **We need people in our lives:** Jennifer Breheny Wallace, *Never Enough* (Portfolio, 2023).

78 **Murthy was quoted:** Leana S. Wen, "The Checkup with Dr. Wen: 8 Ideas from the Surgeon General to Address Loneliness," *Washington Post*, March 9, 2023, washingtonpost.com/opinions/2023/03/09 /surgeon-general-advice-loneliness-isolation.

78 **a "friendship recession":** Daniel A. Cox, "American Men Suffer a Friendship Recession," Survey Center on American Life, July 6, 2021, americansurveycenter.org/commentary/american-men-suffer -a-friendship-recession.

80 **"Being able to feel safe":** Bessel van der Kolk, *The Body Keeps the Score: Brain, Mind, and Body in the Healing of Trauma* (Penguin Books, 2015).

82 **Ginsburg often credited:** Nina Totenberg, "Justice Ruth Bader Ginsburg Reflects on the #MeToo Movement: 'It's About Time,'" NPR, January 22, 2018, npr.org/2018/01/22/579595727/justice -ginsburg-shares-her-own-metoo-story-and-says-it-s-about-time.

82 **"I'm ranked in the top ten":** Rebecca Faye Smith Galli, "Thoughts on Being No One's Number One," *Midlife Boulevard*, May 21, 2017, https://web.archive.org/web/20230321200828/https://midlifeboule vard.com/being-no-ones-number-one

83 **Simone's husband gave Simone:** Simone Gorrindo, *The Wives* (Simon & Schuster, 2024).

88 **"saying yes to ourselves":** Jack Canfield, "Saying NO to others is saying YES to yourself," originally posted on LinkedIn, 2024, linkedin.com/posts/canfieldjack_saying-no-to-others-is-saying -yes-to-yourself-activity-7107727019093749762-Akxf.

Chapter 4: Everyone Needs (to Be) a Cornerman

95 **"secure in the knowledge":** See Jennifer Breheny Wallace, "The Power of Mattering at Work," *Wall Street Journal*, December 1, 2022, wsj.com/articles/the-power-of-mattering-at-work-11669910125.

96 **Researchers call this aspect of mattering:** Nancy K. Schlossberg, "Marginality and Mattering: Key Issues in Building Community,"

New Directions for Student Services, no. 48 (1989): 4, https://doi. org/10.1002/ss.37119894803.

96 **works both ways:** Morris Rosenberg, unpublished manuscript, undated, courtesy of Paul B. Rosenberg, MD.

96 **140 "at-risk" ninth graders:** Cheryl L. Somers, Delila Owens, and Monte Piliawsky, "A Study of High School Dropout Prevention and At-Risk Ninth Graders' Role Models and Motivations for School Completion," *Education* 130, no. 2 (2009): 348.

101 **"The simple power":** John Z., *Grace in Addiction: The Good News of Alcoholics Anonymous for Everybody* (Mockingbird Ministries, 2012).

104 **"I knew what I had to do":** Luke Reddy, "Greatest Fights: Sugar Ray Leonard, Thomas Hearns and 'The Showdown' of 1981," *BBC Sport*, May 8, 2020, bbc.com/sport/boxing/52534002.

107 **"Miscalibrated expectation" is what researchers:** Xuan Zhao and Nicholas Epley, "Surprisingly Happy to Have Helped: Underestimating Prosociality Creates a Misplaced Barrier to Asking for Help," *Psychological Science* 33, no. 10 (2022): 1708–31.

112 **"To get the full value of joy":** Mark Twain, *Following the Equator: A Journey Around the World* (American Publishing Co., 1897), 447.

113 **Neuroimaging studies find:** Sylvia A. Morelli, Matthew D. Sacchet, and Jamil Zaki, "Common and Distinct Neural Correlates of Personal and Vicarious Reward: A Quantitative Meta-Analysis," *NeuroImage* 112 (May 2015): 244–53.

113 **feels authentic delight:** Jeremy Adam Smith, "What Is Sympathetic Joy and How Can You Feel More of It?," *Greater Good Magazine*, March 1, 2022, greatergood.berkeley.edu/article/item /what_is_sympathetic_joy_and_how_can_you_feel_more_of_it.

113 **When feelings of envy:** Jennifer Breheny Wallace, "Put Your Envy to Good Use," *Wall Street Journal*, April 25, 2014, wsj.com/articles /SB10001424052702304279904579517903705459222.

114 **He cofounded Partners In Health:** "The Life of Dr. Paul Farmer," Partners in Health, last updated 2023, pih.org/paul.

114 **philosophy of "accompaniment":** Arthur Kleinman, "Paul Farmer

and the Audacity of Accompaniment," Think Global Health,
February 21, 2024, thinkglobalhealth.org/article/paul-farmer-and
-audacity-accompaniment.

116 **"rather look at the wall"**: Sydney Page, "Former Trash Hauler
Enrolled at Harvard Law Raises $70K for Janitors, Other Workers
There," *Washington Post*, April 15, 2023, washingtonpost.com
/lifestyle/2023/04/15/harvard-law-janitor-rehan-staton.

Chapter 5: Tuning In

124 **"When we attune to others"**: Daniel Siegel, *Mindsight: The New
Science of Personal Transformation* (Random House, 2010).

125 **psychologist Richard Erskine**: Mitchell Kossak, "Attunement and
Free Jazz," *Voices* 8, no. 2 (2008), voices.no/index.php/voices/article
/view/1784/1545.

125 **"Attention is the rarest"**: Simone Weil to Joë Bousquet, April 13,
1942, in *Correspondance*, ed. André A. Devaux (Lausanne: Éditions
L'Âge d'Homme, 1982), 18.

125 **"Still Face" experiment**: Lauren B. Adamson and Janet B. Frick,
"The Still Face: A History of a Shared Experimental Paradigm,"
Infancy 4 (2003): 451–73.

127 **canceling social plans:** "The 2023 Stress in America Survey,"
conducted by the Harris Poll on behalf of the American Psychological
Association, published by the American Psychological Association,
November 2023, 43, apa.org/news/press/releases/stress/2023
/november-2023-topline-data.pdf.

128 **Lucy Lane posted in 2025:** Lydia Patrick, "Millennial Has Important
Message for People Who Cancel Plans Last Minute," *Newsweek*,
February 20, 2025, newsweek.com/millennial-message-cancel-plans
-last-minute-2033088.

129 **"self-imposed solitude"**: Derek Thompson, "The Anti-Social
Century," *The Atlantic*, January 8, 2025, theatlantic.com/magazine
/archive/2025/02/american-loneliness-personality-politics/681091.

131 **an exercise called "mental subtraction"**: For exercises, see

"Mental Subtraction of Relationships: How to Appreciate a Loved One by Imagining Your Life Without Them," available from Greater Good in Action, Greater Good Science Center, ggia.berkeley.edu /practice/mental_subtraction_relationships. For more information on mental subtraction, see Minkyung Koo et al., "It's a Wonderful Life: Mentally Subtracting Positive Events Improves People's Affective States, Contrary to Their Affective Forecasts," *Journal of Personality and Social Psychology* 95, no. 5 (2008): 1217–24.

135 **cause of firefighter deaths:** Miriam Heyman et al., "The Ruderman White Paper on the Mental Health and Suicide of First Responders," Ruderman Family Foundation, April 2018, accessed via Issuu, issuu.com/rudermanfoundation/docs/first_responder _white_paper_final_ac270d530f8bfb.

135 **the nonprofit Chapman Foundation:** For more information on the Chapman Foundation for Caring Communities, see chapmancommunities.org.

136 **"Being heard is so close":** David W. Augsburger, *Caring Enough to Hear and Be Heard: How to Hear and How to Be Heard in Equal Communication* (Ventura, CA: Regal Books, 1982).

138 **the brain's emotion-processing:** Sladjana Lukic et al., "Higher Emotional Granularity Relates to Greater Inferior Frontal Cortex Cortical Thickness in Healthy, Older Adults," *Cognitive, Affective, and Behavioral Neuroscience* 23 (2023): 1401–13.

138 **Yale Center for Emotional Intelligence:** Marc Brackett, "Become an Emotion Scientist in 2023," *Medium*, December 31, 2022, medium .com/@marc.brackett/become-an-emotion-scientist-in-2023 -f2a7408be7ce.

138 **"A real conversation always contains":** David Whyte, "10 Questions That Have No Right to Go Away," *Oprah*, June 15, 2011, oprah.com/oprahs-lifeclass/poet-david-whytes-questions-that -have-no-right-to-go-away_1.

139 **can start to feel:** Juliana Schroeder and Ayelet Fishbach, "Feeling Known Predicts Relationship Satisfaction," *Journal of Experimental Social Psychology* 111 (March 2024).

140 **former FBI hostage negotiator:** Chris Voss (thefbinegotiator), "Why I NEVER Ask 'How Are You?,'" posted on Instagram, 2024, instagram.com/reel/DBw1meXt17P.

142 **"cutting them out":** StoryCorps, "A Moment of Connection, from Opposite Ends of the Political Spectrum," YouTube video, 02:30, from an interview with Amina Amdeen and Joseph Weidknecht, posted by StoryCorps, September 28, 2018, youtube.com/watch?v =91QbjZYSG10.

Chapter 6: When the Rug Gets Pulled

147 **a 1989 academic paper:** Nancy K. Schlossberg, "Marginality and Mattering: Key Issues in Building Community," *New Directions for Student Services*, no. 48 (1989, https://doi.org/10.1002/ss.371198 94803.

148 **cope more creatively:** Rich Feller, "Later Chapters with Nancy Schlossberg," from a series of interviews with National Career Development Association leaders, published by the Association Database, March 1, 2017, associationdatabase.com/aws/NCDA/pt /sd/news_article/135131/_PARENT/OLD_layout_details_cc/false.

149 **"Life is in the transitions":** From an interview with Bruce Feiler. See Nir Eyal, "Handling Life Transitions: Interview with Bruce Feiler," accessed in 2025, nirandfar.com/life-transitions-bruce-feiler.

150 **author Bruce Feiler:** Bruce Feiler, *Life Is in the Transitions: Mastering Change at Any Age* (Penguin Press, 2020).

158 **"the most longed for":** Anatole France, *The Crime of Sylvestre Bonnard* (1881; Modern Library, 1929).

159 **a practical blueprint:** Jordan Deneau, Rylee A. Dionigi, Paula M. van Wyk, and Sean Horton, "Role Models of Aging Among Older Men: Strategies for Facilitating Change and Implications for Health Promotion," *Sports* (Basel, Switzerland) 11, no. 3 (February 2023): 55.

160 **"the beautiful mess effect":** Anna Bruk, Sabine G. Scholl, and Herbert Bless, "Beautiful Mess Effect: Self-Other Differences in Evaluation of Showing Vulnerability," *Journal of Personality and Social Psychology* 115, no. 2 (2018): 192–205.

161 **"two ways of spreading light"**: Edith Wharton, "Vesalius in Zante," *North American Review* 174, no. 552 (1902): 625–31.

161 **In Senegal, a highly regarded value:** Ebrima Sall, "Nio ko Bokk, a Philosophy of Giving," published by Trust Africa, 2024, trustafrica.org/wp-content/uploads/2024/07/17.-Nio-ko-Bokk-a-Philosophy-of-Giving.pdf.

165 **rising "deaths of despair"**: Anne Case and Angus Deaton, *Deaths of Despair and the Future of Capitalism* (Princeton, NJ: Princeton University Press, 2020).

165 **One study on suicidal ideation:** Fiona L. Shand et al., "What Might Interrupt Men's Suicide? Results from an Online Survey of Men," *BMJ Open* 5, no. 10 (October 2015).

165 **Economists at Goldman Sachs:** Jan Hatzius et al., "The Potentially Large Effects of Artificial Intelligence on Economic Growth," *Goldman Sachs Economic Research* (March 2023), goldmansachs.com/insights/articles/generative-ai-could-raise-global-gdp-by-7-percent.

165 **Technology leaders like Bill Gates:** Tom Huddleston Jr., "Bill Gates: Within 10 Years, AI Will Replace Many Doctors and Teachers—Humans Won't Be Needed 'For Most Things,'" CNBC, March 26, 2025, cnbc.com/2025/03/26/bill-gates-on-ai-humans-wont-be-needed-for-most-things.html.

166 **"even a little bit scary"**: Olivia Farrar, "Bill Gates on AI and Innovation," *Harvard Magazine*, February 4, 2025, updated February 14, 2025, harvardmagazine.com/2025/02/harvard-bill-gates-ai-and-innovation.

170 **called regenerative farming:** *Kiss the Ground*, directed by Joshua Tickell and Rebecca Harrell Tickell (Big Picture Ranch, The Redford Center, and Benenson Productions, 2020).

Chapter 7: How We Spend Our Days

174 **As I listened to:** Annie Dillard, *The Writing Life* (New York: HarperCollins, 1989).

174 **US employee engagement:** Gallup Workplace, "What Is Employee

Engagement, and How Do You Improve It?," Gallup, accessed June 2025, gallup.com/workplace/285674/improve-employee-engagement-workplace.aspx.

174 **Two-thirds of employees worldwide:** "Indicators: Employee Wellbeing," Gallup, accessed June 2025, gallup.com/394424/indicator-employee-wellbeing.aspx.

174 **"humans are machines":** Dale Whelehan, "Something curious has been happening inside me since the election of the new Pope," originally published on LinkedIn, May 2025, linkedin.com/feed/update/urn:li:activity:7326589036377092096.

175 **200 percent of their salary:** Corey Tatel and Ben Wigert, "42% of Employee Turnover Is Preventable but Often Ignored," Gallup Workplace, July 10, 2024, gallup.com/workplace/646538/employee-turnover-preventable-often-ignored.aspx.

175 **article titled "'Everybody's Replaceable'":** Chip Cutter, "'Everybody's Replaceable': The New Ways Bosses Talk About Workers," *Wall Street Journal*, May 11, 2025, wsj.com/lifestyle/workplace/corporate-bosses-workers-culture-changing-cbd19c2c.

175 **A 2025 leadership survey:** "Global Leadership Forecast 2025," Development Dimensions International, 2025, media.ddiworld.com/research/global-leadership-forecast-2025-report.pdf.

179 **"they don't care what you think":** Gordon L. Flett et al., "The Anti-Mattering Scale: Development, Psychometric Properties and Associations with Well-Being and Distress Measures in Adolescents and Emerging Adults," *Journal of Psychoeducational Assessment* 40, no. 1 (2021): 37–59.

180 **made other egregious errors:** Jennifer Breheny Wallace, "The Costs of Workplace Rudeness: Uncivil Behavior at Work Takes a Real Toll on Employees, Research Finds," *Wall Street Journal*, August 18, 2017, wsj.com/articles/the-costs-of-workplace-rudeness-1503061187.

180 **Anti-mattering impacts decision-making:** Arieh Riskin et al., "The Impact of Rudeness on Medical Team Performance: A Randomized Trial," *Pediatrics* 136, no. 3 (2015): 487–95.

180 **highly engaged teams:** Katelyn Hedrick, Ben Wigert, and Ryan

Pendell, "Despite Employer Prioritization, Employee Wellbeing Falters," Gallup Workplace, November 4, 2024, gallup.com /workplace/652769/despite-employer-prioritization-employee -wellbeing-falters.aspx.

181 **the 100 Best Companies double:** Ted Kitterman, "When Employees Thrive, Companies More Than Triple Their Stock Market Performance," Great Place to Work, April 2, 2025, web .archive.org/web/20250813074108/https://www.greatplacetowork .com/resources/blog/when-employees-thrive-companies-triple -their-stock-market-performance.

185 **"Far and away the best":** Theodore Roosevelt, *The Key to Success in Life* (Federated Publishing, 1916), 12, Theodore Roosevelt Birthplace National Historic Site, Theodore Roosevelt Digital Library, Dickinson State University, theodorerooseveltcenter.org /Research/Digital-Library/Record?libID=o283099.

186 **speaking with scholarship recipients:** Adam M. Grant, "Outsource Inspiration," forthcoming in *Putting Positive Leadership in Action*, edited by J. E. Dutton and G. Spreitzer, faculty.wharton.upenn.edu/wp-content/uploads/2013/12/Grant _OutsourceInspiration.pdf.

188 **the famous Hawthorne Studies:** Morris Rosenberg, unpublished manuscript, undated, courtesy of Paul B. Rosenberg, MD, 8.

190 **have termed "Fast Friends":** Arthur Aron et al., "The Experimental Generation of Interpersonal Closeness: A Procedure and Some Preliminary Findings," *Personality and Social Psychology Bulletin* 23 (1997): 363–77.

191 **increasingly meaningful prompts:** "36 Questions for Increasing Closeness," Greater Good in Action, Greater Good Science Center, accessed June 2025, ggia.berkeley.edu/practice/36_questions_for _increasing_closeness.

191 **significantly lower turnover:** Ruth Gotian, "The Overlooked Way to Reduce Employee Turnover by 59%," *Forbes*, April 19, 2022, forbes.com/sites/ruthgotian/2022/04/19/the-overlooked-way-to -reduce-employee-turnover-by-59.

194 **Managers with high emotional intelligence:** "Tools for Measuring

Emotional Intelligence in Your Workforce," LeaderFactor, January 27, 2025, leaderfactor.com/learn/measuring-emotional-intelligence.

195 **Or Austin, who started:** "Careers: The Best Team on the Planet, Always," Jersey Mike's Subs, accessed June 2025, jerseymikes.com /careers.

196 **a 2021 Pew Research study:** Kim Parker and Juliana Menasce Horowitz, "Majority of Workers Who Quit a Job in 2021 Cite Low Pay, No Opportunities for Advancement, Feeling Disrespected," Pew Research Center, March 9, 2022, pewresearch.org/short-reads /2022/03/09/majority-of-workers-who-quit-a-job-in-2021-cite-low -pay-no-opportunities-for-advancement-feeling-disrespected.

197 **they plan to stay:** "Workplace Learning for Better Performance and Stronger People," Gallup Learning, accessed June 2025, gallup .com/learning/home.aspx.

198 **"Work, among all its abstracts":** David Whyte, "Work," in *Consolations: The Solace, Nourishment and Underlying Meaning of Everyday Words* (Many Rivers Press, 2021).

199 **Grant's research reveals:** Knowledge at Wharton Staff, "Givers vs. Takers: The Surprising Truth About Who Gets Ahead," Knowledge at Wharton Podcast, April 10, 2013, knowledge.wharton.upenn .edu/podcast/knowledge-at-wharton-podcast/givers-vs-takers-the -surprising-truth-about-who-gets-ahead.

201 **overlooked, micromanaged, or excluded:** Jamie Ducharme, "Work Is the New Doctor's Office," *Time*, January 3, 2024, time .com/6548866/how-work-affects-your-health.

201 **"the spillover-crossover model":** Arnold B. Bakker and Evangelia Demerouti, "The Spillover-Crossover Model," in *New Frontiers in Work and Family Research*, ed. Sandra L. Blithe and Joseph G. Grzywacz (New York: Psychology Press, 2013). Katie M. Lawson et al., "Daily Positive Spillover and Crossover from Mothers' Work to Youth Health," *Journal of Family Psychology* 28, no. 6 (2014): 897–907.

202 **into their personal relationships:** "State of the Global Workplace: Understanding Employees, Informing Leaders, 2025 Report," Gallup, 2025, gallup.com/workplace/349484/state-of-the-global-workplace .aspx.

202 **Some scholars:** Carole Pateman, *Participation and Democratic Theory* (Cambridge: Cambridge University Press, 1970); Irma Rybnikova, "Spillover Effect of Workplace Democracy: A Conceptual Revision," *Frontiers in Psychology* 13 (2022): 933263.

Chapter 8: Be an Architect

207 **According to the Survey Center:** Daniel A. Cox et al., "Public Places and Commercial Spaces: How Neighborhood Amenities Foster Trust and Connection in American Communities," Survey Center on American Life, October 20, 2021, americansurveycenter.org /research/public-places-and-commercial-spaces-how-neighborhood -amenities-foster-trust-and-connection-in-american-communities.

207 **"Americans with less access":** Daniel A. Cox and Sam Pressler, "Disconnected: The Growing Class Divide in American Civic Life," Survey Center on American Life, August 22, 2024, americansurveycenter.org/research/disconnected-places-and-spaces.

208 **"We need to understand *where*":** *Connective Tissue* and Sam Pressler, "How to Think Structurally About Connection Within Communities," *Connective Tissue* newsletter via Substack, January 11, 2024, connectivetissue.substack.com/p/how-to-think-structurally -about-connection.

209 **"Do your little bit":** Richard Branson, "Remembering Archbishop Desmond Tutu," Richard Branson's Blog, Virgin, December 26, 2021, virgin.com/branson-family/richard-branson-blog/remembering -archbishop-desmond-tutu.

210 **Copenhagen's busy streets:** "Jan Gehl," Project for Public Spaces, December 31, 2008, pps.org/article/jgehl.

210 **"We shape our buildings":** "House of Commons Rebuilding," UK Parliament debate, October 28, 1943, api.parliament.uk/historic -hansard/commons/1943/oct/28/house-of-commons-rebuilding.

211 **Patty Smith and her husband:** Patty Smith, "Stoop Coffee: How a Simple Idea Transformed My Neighborhood," *Supernuclear* via Substack, March 25, 2025, supernuclear.substack.com/p/stoop -coffee-how-a-simple-idea-transformed.

211 **Lisa and Mark Walter:** S. Jason Cole, "'Paint Your Dot': Burton Reminds Residents of Their Role in the Bigger Picture," *Excelsior Citizen*, March 30, 2025, excelsiorcitizen.com/paint-your-dot -burton-reminds-residents-of-their-role-in-the-bigger-picture.

211 **The Walters bought two flamingos:** Justin Meyer, "What Is Flamingo Friday?," The Popular Flamingo, February 3, 2023, thepopularflamingo.com/blogs/posts/what-is-flamingo-friday.

212 **Only 4.1 percent:** "American Time Use Survey," Bureau of Labor Statistics, 2023, bls.gov/tus/tables/a2-2023.pdf; Ellen Cushing, "Americans Need to Party More," *The Atlantic*, January 4, 2025, https://www.theatlantic.com/family/archive/2025/01/throw-more -parties-loneliness/681203/.

213 **When Alex Hoskyn had:** Alexandra Hoskyn, "Connecting in Cafes," TedXKazimierzWomen via TED, December 2019, ted.com/talks /alexandra_hoskyn_connecting_in_cafes.

214 **story of Joan and Sarah:** Hoskyn, "Connecting in Cafes."

215 **"the mere exposure effect":** Rocco Palumbo et al., "When Twice Is Better than Once: Increased Liking of Repeated Items Influences Memory in Younger and Older Adults," *BMC Psychology* 9 (2021).

216 **warmth of a hand:** "Oxytocin: The Love Hormone," Harvard Health Publishing, Harvard Medical School, last updated 2025, health.harvard.edu/mind-and-mood/oxytocin-the-love-hormone.

216 **college dorm friendships:** Kristina Borrman, "Studying Friendship in Housing the MIT School of Architecture at MIT in the Postwar Years," *Journal of Urban History* 48, no. 5 (2020): 1100–1120.

217 **acts as a "social glue":** Kaitlin Woolley and Sarah Lim, "Interpersonal Consequences of Joint Food Consumption for Connection and Conflict," *Social and Personal Psychology Compass* (2023): e12748.

217 **meals over a campfire:** Jan-Emmanuel De Neve et al., "Sharing Meals with Others: How Sharing Meals Supports Happiness and Social Connections," *World Happiness Report*, 2025, worldhappiness .report/ed/2025/sharing-meals-with-others-how-sharing-meals -supports-happiness-and-social-connections/.

218 **"the soup suppers":** Kathy Gunst, "Soup Party: A Potluck Gathering,"

NewEngland.com Magazine, March 11, 2014, newengland.com
/today/soup-party.

218 **Play, studies find:** Gillian M. Sandstrom, Erica J. Boothby, and
Gus Cooney, "Talking to Strangers: A Week-Long Intervention
Reduces Psychological Barriers to Social Connection," *Journal of
Experimental Social Psychology* 102 (September 2022): 104356.

219 **face-to-face connection:** Dodai Stewart, "New York City's Hottest
Hangout Is a 500-Person Board Game Night," *New York Times*,
April 19, 2025, https://www.nytimes.com/2025/04/19/nyregion
/new-york-city-giant-game-night.html.

220 **In response to growing loneliness:** "Jumbo Opens 'Chat Checkouts'
to Combat Loneliness Among the Elderly," *Dutch News*, September 28,
2021, dutchnews.nl/2021/09/jumbo-opens-chat-checkouts-to
-combat-loneliness-among-the-elderly.

223 **Drawing on therapy-informed:** Justin Adam Gelzhiser and
Lorenzo Lewis, "Black Barbers as Mental Health Advocates, and
Interpersonal Violence and Suicide Preventors in the Local
Community," *Mental Health & Prevention* 31 (September 2023):
200291.

224 **Today, the Confess Project:** For more information, see
theconfessprojectofamerica.org.

225 **"Stewardship of the space":** Yasmeen Abdallah, "More than a Place
to Read: Memphis Library's Innovative Transformation," *The Urban
Activist*, February 8, 2022, theurbanactivist.com/culture/more
-than-a-place-to-read-memphis-librarys-innovative-transformation.

Epilogue

229 **"No one is finally dead":** Terry Pratchett, *Reaper Man* (Harper,
2013).

231 **We want to know that:** Jennifer Breheny Wallace, "Mattering in
the Modern World," TED, September 2025.

Index

Accenture, 199
accepting investment,
    102–5
accompaniment, 114–15
accountability
    ego extension and, 96
    envy and, 113
achievement, 3
Achilles International, 110
acts of kindness, 54–57
adding value, 4, 39
Adler, Alfred, 6
advice-giving effect, 46
Aging Rebels, 167–69, 171
agricultural practices, 163–64,
    169–71
ahimsa, 56
air pollution, 170
alcohol-related deaths, 10
Ali, Muhammad, 103
Amdeen, Amina, 142

American Psychological
    Association, 127
Anglesea Arms, 204
anticipated transitions, 148–49
anti-mattering, 10–11, 179
    impacts of, 180
    moments of, 177
    "taker" mindset and, 198
anxiety, 3, 5, 60, 75, 193
appreciation
    impact file and, 27
    notes of, 118
    qualities of person and impact
        of, 23–24
    Wall of Appreciation, 185
Archer, Colton, 44–45
Archer Cleaners, 44
Aristotle, 6
article clubs, 219
artificial intelligence, 162, 165–66
    generative, 175

Index

Ashworth, Donna, 31
asking what is needed, 50–52
atman, 6
attention, 10, 126
  defining, 124–25
  fine-tuning, 132
attunement, 121, 123, 124,
  237–39
  breaks in, 126
  bridging divides and, 141–42
  broadcasting, 133–37
  disconnection from emotions
    and, 137
  emotional, 132
  emotions and, 126
  fighting inertia and, 127–30
  modeling, 140–41
  naming needs and, 141
  organizational success and, 194
  practicing, 126–27
  to self, 137–38
  teaching, 135–36
  work and, 183
Augsburger, David W., 136
Authentic Connections
  Groups, 76
authentic relationships, 76
automation, job losses from, 165

bailing, 127
Baldwin, James, 74
Banana Cabaret comedy club, 205
Barbershop Books, 222
barbershops, 222–24
Barry-Wehmiller, 194–95

Bates Trucking & Trash
  Removal, 117
beautiful mess effect, 160–61
Bedford (pub), 203–9, 218, 225–26
belonging, 5
benign envy, 113
biodiversity, 170
board game cafés, 218–19
board game nights, 218
book clubs, 79, 80, 219
Boston Marathon, 110–12
boundaries, 72
Bowie State University, 97, 119
Brackett, Marc, 138
brain cancer, 36
bridging divides, 141–42
broadcasting back, 133–37
broadcasting out, 136
Brody, Lauren Smith, 27
Brown, Louise, 49
Bulanow, Greg, 15–25, 28, 31–33,
  133–37
Bureau of Labor Statistics, 212
burnout, 5, 9, 174, 176
  connection reducing, 76
  lack of importance and, 64–65
  leaders and, 175
  purpose and, 17
Burton, David, 212–13
Butler, Sean, 163–64, 169–71
butterfly effect, 55
BW Papersystems, 183–84

canceling, 127, 129
cancer, 36, 108, 144

care, 3
caregivers, 65
 connection and, 77
 overwhelm in, 67
 resilience of, 76
Case, Anne, 165
casual hangouts, 80
change, 145–46
 categories of, 148–49
 large-scale, 162–64
 mattering after, 147–49
 mattering lens, 153–55
Chapman, Bob, 195
Chapman Foundation for Caring
 Communities, 135
chatty cafés, 214
childcare, 66
Churchill, Winston, 210
City Girls Who Walk, 50
civic infrastructure, 208
clean fuel, 179
climate change, 164
Code Lavender, 87
colon cancer, 144
community
 fighting friendship recession
  and, 78–80
 invisibility and, 19
 mattering and, 5–7
 mattering core and, 12–13
 pub's roles in, 203–4
 reciprocity effect and, 116–18
 sharing information and, 47
 stewardship of, 224–26
 as transactions, 66–67

compassion, 3, 55–56
Confess Project, 223–24
connecting
 authentic relationships and, 76
 burnout reduction through, 76
 of colleagues with impact,
  183–86
 to impact, 26
 isolation and, 129
 before leaving for day, 85
 stress reduction through, 76
coping strategies
 me-search and, 159
 transitions and, 157–58
 unhealthy, 133
cornermen, 102, 103–5, 119
 being, 108–9
 finding, 105–8
 offering time, talent, and
  treasure, 109–12
 transitions and, 152
cortisol, 76
COVID-19, 44, 162, 205
culture of mattering, 180, 181
culture wars, 9
curiosity, 159–60
Cushing, Ellen, 212

dads' groups, 79
daily walks, 73
deaths of despair, 10, 165
Deaton, Angus, 165
decision-making, anti-mattering
 impact on, 180
depression, 3, 9

detachment, 19
details, mattering and, 84–86
Dillard, Annie, 174
Dillon, Matt, 222
dirty fuel, 179
disabled athletes, 110
disconnection, 5, 9–13, 18
    from emotions, 137
disengagement, 174–76
dismissiveness, 179
disruptive events, 150
donations, 37–38
Drury, Chuck, 196–98
Drury Hotels, 196–98
Dundee, Angelo, 103–5

ego extension, 91, 96, 114, 124,
    237–39
    work and, 183
Electrical Contractors Association
    of Western Pennsylvania, 187
emergency financial support, 197
emotional attunement, 132
emotional intelligence, 138
    leadership and, 194
emotional resilience, 133, 137
emotions
    attunement and, 126
    disconnection from, 137
    noticing clues of, 139
    workplace and, 194
emotion scientist, 138–40
empathetic listening, 223
Empire Board Game Library, 218
employee engagement, 174

endometriosis, 49
energy, 39–40
engagement, 176
    employee, 174
    work performance and, 180
environmental policies, 166, 170
envy, 113
Erikson, Erik, 196
Erskine, Richard, 125
eudaimonia, 6
European Union, 170
existential reliance, 56

families
    spouses as scaffolding of, 69
    as villages, 66
Farmer, Paul, 114
farming, 163–64, 169–71
Fast Friends, 190–91
feedback, 20, 22, 25, 97
    asking for help and, 107
    to leaders, 188–89
    as love language, 105
feeling valued, 4
Feiler, Bruce, 149, 150
Feiner, Paul, 51
Fifth Trimester, 27
fighting inertia, attunement and,
    127–30
firefighting, 16
    feedback in, 20–21
    invisibility and, 17–20
    patient outcome follow-up
        and, 20
    routine and, 25

seeing impact of work and,
    17–18
sense of detachment and, 19
suicide and, 135
fire investigations, 20–21
Fiverr, 175
Fix IT! Greenburgh (app), 51
flaking, 127
Flamingo Friday, 211
Flett, Gordon, 10, 63, 95
follow-up systems, 20–21, 25
food
    agricultural practices and, 164,
        169–70
    open-kitchen restaurants
        and, 29
    as social glue, 217–18
food banks, 47
food insecurity, 60
Fortune 100 Best Companies to
    Work For, 180–81
France, Anatole, 158
friendship recession, fighting,
    78–81
fuel, 179

Gallup
    on disengagement, 174–75
    on employee sense of
        mattering, 180
Gates, Bill, 165–66
Gehl, Jan, 210
generative AI, 175
generativity, 196
Georgia-Pacific, 44

gestures
    acts of kindness as, 54–56
    of recognition, 19–20, 131–32
Ginsburg, Marty, 82
Ginsburg, Ruth Bader, 82
giver mindset, 199
glioblastoma, 36
Global Financial Crisis of
    2008, 162
Glue Award, 28
GoFundMe, 19
golden rule, 52
Goldman Sachs, 165
Good Samaritan story, 56
Gorrindo, Simone, 68–70, 74–75,
    81, 83–84
Grant, Adam, 186, 198–99
Grant, Heidi, 46
gratitude
    journal of, 27
    messages of, 30–31
Great Place to Work, 180, 188
Greenburgh, New York, 51

Hallman, Shamichael, 224–25
Happy Teacher Revolution
    group, 89
hardship
    accompanying others in,
        114–15
    assistance programs for
        financial, 197
Harvard Law School, 101, 108,
    116–18
Hawthorne Studies, 188

Index

Hearns, Tommy, 104
help
   accepting, 106–7
   inviting, 46–47
helpers, support for, 77
helper's high, 39
Hoskyn, Alex, 213–14
hospitality, therapeutic work
   through, 206
hospitals
   codes, 87
   privacy laws and, 134
Hughes, John, 192–93
Huskey, Jake, 194–95

identity
   loss of, 8, 36
   me-search and, 171
   narrowing of, 69
   other's growth and, 114
   redefining roles and, 169–72
   retirement and, 157–58
   transitions and, 146, 147,
      150, 151
   work and, 165
identity crisis, retirement and, 157
imago Dei, 6
impact
   connecting colleagues with,
      183–86
   connecting to, 26
   disconnection from, 18–19
   greater, connecting to, 29
   notes about, 30
   seeing, of work, 17–18

impact files, 27–28
importance, 59, 63, 237–38
   feeling a sense of, 64–65, 82
   of in-person interaction,
      127–28
   invisibility and, 68–70
   work and, 183
"I'm telling" initiative, 20–24, 28
inertia
   breaking through, 231
   social, 127–30
information, sharing, 46–47
INNTouch, 197
in-person interaction, importance
   of, 127–28
insomnia, 50
inspiration
   others' success as, 113
   role models and, 159
Instagram, 50
internalizing disregard, 97
investment
   accepting, 102–5
   in employees, 195–200
   joy in others' success and, 114
   mutual, 211
invisibility, 17–20, 94
   anti-mattering and, 179
   importance and, 68–70
invisible support, 115
invitations, 160–62
inviting help, 46–47
in vitro fertilization (IVF), 49
isolation, 128–29
IVF. *See* in vitro fertilization

James, William, 22
Jersey Mike's, 192–93, 195
job losses, 165
    reducing impact of, 166
Johnson, Kelli, 220–21
Jones, Chad, 186–87
Joy (film), 49
joy, sharing, 112–14
just transitions, 164–67

karama, 6
Karp, Michael, 167
karuna, 56
Katie, 103, 108–9
Kaufman, Micha, 175
kindness
    acts of, 54–57
    moments of, 54
Kiss the Ground
    (documentary), 170
Koch, Laurie, 189
Kohn, Brianna, 50
Kolk, Bessel van der, 80
Kundera, Milan, 41

labor unions, 166
Lane, Lucy, 128
large-scale changes, 162–64
laundromats, 219–20
leaders
    burnout and, 175
    feedback to, 188–89
leadership
    connecting work to impact
        and, 185

emotional intelligence and, 194
    mattering and, 181
leadership training, 176
leaning into strengths, 44–46
Leonard, Sugar Ray, 103–5
"Let's Go Fly a Kite" (song), 59
Lewis, Lorenzo, 222–24
libraries, 224–25
life expectancy, 9
Life Is in the Transitions
    (Feiler), 150
lifequakes, 150
life transitions, 145–46, 151
    cornermen and, 152
    curiosity and, 159–60
    major, 150
    mattering lens, 153–55
    me-search and, 155–60
lighting, 188
limits, protecting, 86–88
little contributions notes, 27
logging, 165
loneliness, 8, 9, 80
    Murthy on combating, 78
    paying attention to, 50
    in relationships, 130–31
long arm of the job, 201–2
loss, 227–28
love
    doing small things with great,
        54–57
    passion tax and, 70
love language, feedback as, 105
Luthar, Suniya, 76
Lütke, Tobi, 175

Index

Mahoney, Julie Plaut, 35–39, 41, 53, 54, 57, 83, 86–87

Making Caring Common, 67

malicious envy, 113

Mangione, Pietro, 199–200

martyrdom, 61, 71

Mary Poppins (film), 59, 89

matchmaking, 47–49

mattering, 229
  business case for, 178–82
  after changes, 147–49
  community and, 5–7
  culture of, 180, 181
  defining, 4
  defining spaces for, 210–15
  details and, 84–86
  erosion of, at work, 173–74
  leading with, 181
  as meta-need, 5
  modern crisis of, 7–11
  moments of, 177
  nudges for, 220–21
  as practice, 12
  retirement and, 155–60
  scaffolding spaces for, 217–19
  scale, 222–24
  to self, 70–73
  self-assessment of, 237–39
  work and, 165
  workplace and, 201–2

mattering core, 11–14
  at work, 182–83

mattering lens, 153–55

mattering practices, rituals as, 6–7

mattering space
  committing to, 215–17
  defining, 210–15
  not from scratch, 220–21
  scaffolding for, 217–19
  stewardship of, 224–26

Mayo Clinic, 76

McLeod, Erin, 167

meeting needs, 42–44

mental health
  Code Lavender and, 87
  overwhelm and, 67
  teacher, 88–89

mental subtraction, 131

mentorship, 196, 199

mere exposure effect, 215–16

me-search, 155–60, 171

messages of gratitude, 184–85

micromanagement, 191

Midlife Boulevard (magazine), 82

military spouses, 68–69

misattunement, 126

miscalibrated expectation, 107

moai groups, 78

modeling attunement, 140–41

morale
  firefighters and, 16–17
  Hawthorne Studies and, 188

lack of closure and, 18

Mother Teresa, 56

mudita, 113

Murphy, Hope, 218

Murthy, Vivek, 78, 81

mutual investment, 211

naming needs, 141
NASA, janitor at, 28–29
National Center for Education
 Statistics, 96
National Health Service, 205
needs
 meeting, 42–44
 naming, 141
negativity bias, 27
neighbors
 being matchmaker with,
  47–48
 childcare and, 66
 leaning into strengths and,
  44–45
 trust in, 9
Newton at Home, 37, 38
Nextdoor, 79
nonevent events, 149
nonprofits, 38
 connecting impact to work at,
  184–85
 trust and, 54
nonverbal communication, 223
notes of appreciation, 118
noticing one small thing,
 24–26

obligation, 40
open-kitchen restaurants, 29
organic farming, 169–71
organizational success,
 attunement and, 194
Our Community Listens, 135
ovarian cancer, 108

overdoses, 10
overwhelm, 63
 in caregivers, 67
 mental health and, 67
oxytocin, 216

pain
 anti-mattering and, 10–11
 of dismissal, 94–95
 recognition of, 124
 using as compass, 49–50
Paralympics, 110
parenting
 coping with demands of, 73
 life transitions and, 148
 standards of, 65–66
parents, death of, 227, 230
Partners in Health, 114
part of bigger whole, 28–30
party deficit, 212
passion tax, 70
pay-to-play village, 65–68
Peckler, Mindy Frankel, 37, 38,
 53, 83
personalizing support, 192–95
personal optimization, 70
personal policies, 88
pet adoption, 42
Pew Research, 66
 on reasons for quitting, 196
platinum rule, 52
play, 218
positive communication, 223
poverty, 60
Pratchett, Terry, 230

Index

President's Council (Drury Hotels initiative), 197
Pressler, Sam, 208
prestige, 10
Prilleltensky, Isaac, 63
prioritizing, 89
    being prioritized, 63–64
    each other, 73–75
    self, 71–73
    taking turns in, 81–84
productivity, Hawthorne Studies and, 188
protecting limits, 86–88
proximal separation, 201
psychological checkups, 135
PTSD, 135
public spaces, 204
pub ministry, 209
pub therapy, 206, 209
Purdy, Jean, 49
purpose, 5, 17
    being part of whole and, 28

quiet quitting, 174
quitting, advancement opportunities and, 196

random acts of kindness, 55
reciprocity effect, 116–19
recognition, 3, 15, 64, 124, 237–38
    encouraging, 21–22
    gestures of, 19–20, 131–32
    work and, 182
redefining roles, 169–72
red flag emoji, 141

regenerative farming, 170, 171
relationships
    authentic, 76
    building deeper, 75–78
    loneliness in, 130–31
    maintenance of, 77–78
    taking turns in, 81–84
reliance, 35, 124, 237–38
    culture of self, 66
    existential, 56
    fostering through trust, 52–54
    work and, 182, 186–89
religion
    mattering in, 6
    turning away from, 9
remote work, 42–43, 173, 191
Repair Café, 47–48
repetition
    committing to space and, 215
    group formation and, 78
    trust and, 52
resilience
    caregiver, 76
    emotional, 133, 137
    mattering core and, 12
responsibility, 40, 42
responsibility to others, 40
retirement, 155–60, 173
    identity and, 157–58
rituals, 132
    as mattering practices, 6–7
role models, transitions and, 159
roles
    loss of, 147–49
    redefining, 169–72

Index

Rook & Pawn, 218

Roosevelt, Theodore, 185

Rosenberg, Morris, 5, 19, 96

Rosten, Leo, 49

Rotary clubs, 213

routine

    firefighting and, 25

    volunteering and, 54

rudeness, 179–80

Salerno, Joelle, 186–88

scaffolding, 217–19

scale mattering, 222–24

Schlossberg, Nancy, 145–49, 151, 155–59, 167–69, 171–73

school-dropout rates, tutoring and, 96

school supplies, 47

Schumacher, Jason, 188–89

self

    attunement to, 137–38

    mattering to, 70–73

    others' role in sense of, 125

    prioritizing, 71–73

self-care, 70, 72, 89

self-harm, 11

self-isolation, 128–29

self-reflection, 176

self-reliance, 66, 77

    finding cornermen and, 106

self-sufficiency, 19

Senior Friendship Centers, 167

September 11, 2001, terrorist attacks, 162

shame, misattunement and, 126

sharing information, 46–47

sharing joy, 112–14

Shaw, George Bernard, 11

Shepard, Alexis, 72

Shopify, 175

Siegel, Dan, 124

60 Minutes (television show), 102–3, 106

skill building, 176

slow checkout lanes, 221

small things with great love, 54–57

Smith, Patty, 211

Snakes & Lattes, 218

social farming, 171

social glue, 217

social health crisis, 10

social inertia, 127–30

social interactions, 216

    third spaces and, 207

social media, 9, 89, 128

social networking apps, 79

social networks, 31

social supports

    as transactions, 66–67

    transitions and, 146

social time, compression of, 216

Sofa Super Store fire, 32–33

soil microbiome, 170

S&P 500, 181

spaces

    committing to, 215–17

    defining, 210–15

    for mattering, 210–15

    reciprocal relationships to, 210

    scaffolding for, 217–19

spillover-crossover model, 201
spouses
    military, 68, 69
    protecting time for, 77
    as scaffolding of families, 69
stagnation, 196
Staton, Rehan, 91–94, 97–103,
        107–8, 116–19
stewards, 224–26
"Still Face" experiment, 125–26,
        129–30
story cards, 183–84
strengths, leaning into,
        44–46
stress
    connection reducing, 76
    spilling over from work to
        personal, 201
substance use, 11
suicidal ideation, 165
suicides, 10, 135
support
    invisible, 115
    layers of, 135–36
    personalizing, 192–95
    surprise, 115
support staff, interacting with,
        116–19
surprise support, 115
Survey Center on American
        Life, 207

table talk, 217
"taker" mindset, 198–99
taking turns, 81–84

Taskrabbit, 67
teacher mental health, 88–89
Teach for America, 60
teaching, 59–62
technology
    in-person interactions and, 9
    interaction replaced by, 48
television production, 102–3
teranga, 161
texting, 127, 128, 216
thank-you notes, 27, 53
therapeutic work, through
        hospitality, 206
third spaces, 9
    finding, 207–10
    social interactions and, 207
Thomas, Danna, 59–63, 70–71,
        74, 81, 87–90
Thompson, Derek, 129
three T's (time, talent, and
        treasure), 109–12
tikkun olam ("repairing the
        world"), 55
TikTok, 50
time
    childcare and, 66
    compression of social, 216
    cornermen and, 109–12
    protecting, for spouses, 77
    volunteering and sense of,
        39–40
time, talent, and treasure (three
        T's), 109–12
toxic workplaces, 186
"traffic BFF" ritual, 44

transactions, social supports as, 66–67

transitions, 145
cornermen and, 152
curiosity and, 159–60
identity and, 146, 147, 150, 151
invitations and, 160–62
just, 164–67
major, 150
mattering lens, 153–55
me-search and, 155–60
social supports and, 146
steps to take during, 152–53

transition theory, 148–49

Trek Bikes, 188–89

Tronick, Edward, 125–26

trophies, 28

trust
fostering reliance through, 52–54
in neighbors, 9
nonprofits and, 54
repetition and, 52
volunteering and, 53
workplaces and, 186–88

tuning in, 123–27, 130–33, 142
to self, 137–38

turning outward, 38–41

tutoring, 93, 97
dropout rates and, 96

Tutu, Desmond, 209

Twain, Mark, 112

UBI. *See* universal basic income

unanticipated transitions, 149

United Auto Workers, 145

universal basic income (UBI), 166

University of Maryland, 97

updating titles, 167–69

US Army, 68–69

video calls, 127

village
family as, 66
pay-to-play, 65–68

volunteering, 39–40, 57
protecting limits and, 86–87
strengths and, 45
trust and, 53

Vonnegut, Kurt, 43

Voss, Chris, 140–41

vulnerability, 61

Wackman, John, 47–48

Walker, Abraham, 79, 81

Wall of Appreciation, 185

Wall Street Journal, The (newspaper), 103, 175

Walter, Lisa, 211

Walter, Mark, 211

Washroom, 220–21

water pollution, 170

water runoff, 170

Wednesday Breakfast Club, 122, 143–44

Weidknecht, Joseph, 142

weightlessness, 37

Weil, Simone, 125

Index

Welcome Home, 38, 53, 54, 57, 83, 86

well-being
    mattering and, 5
    meaningful contribution and, 6
    pleasure in other's, 113
    prioritizing, 189–92
    volunteering and, 39
Western Electric, 188
Wharton, Edith, 161
Whelehan, Dale, 174
whole, part of bigger, 28–30
Whyte, David, 139, 198
Widener, Bill, 29
Winckowski, Peggy, 121–23, 128, 143–44, 214
Winckowski, Sam, 122, 143–44
Winfrey, Oprah, 18
wisdom
    parents sharing, 66
    sharing, 46
The Wives (Gorrindo), 84
work
    attunement and, 183
    connecting colleagues with impact, 183–86
    ego extension and, 183
    engagement and performance in, 180
    erosion of mattering in, 173–74
    identity and, 165

impact and, 183–86
importance and, 183
mattering and, 165
mattering core at, 182–83
prioritizing well-being and, 189–92
recognition and, 182
reliance and, 182, 186–89
seeing impact of, 17–18
stress spilling over from, 201
workplaces, 9
    advancement opportunities in, 196
    business case for mattering and, 178–82
    disconnection from impact in, 18
    emotions and, 194
    employee engagement in, 174
    investing in employees, 195–200
    mattering and, 201–2
    personalizing support in, 192–95
    "taker" and "giver" mindsets and, 198–99
    toxic, 186
    trust and, 186–88

zakat, 56
Zoom, 42, 190